To Suzanne,

My lovely friend of the bees....

I'd like to meet you in a timeless, placeless, place

Somewhere out of context and beyond all consequences

Suzanne Vega, Language

Introduction

Orthodox medicine deals in exact and measurable science. It has no place for symbolic connections. But the mind body spirit connection of alternative medicine makes it necessary to investigate how these symbolic truths affect how we feel...because ultimately those resulting emotions profoundly influence our physical wellness too.

There is no deeper running symbol than that of the rose (except perhaps the shape of a heart or the cross, maybe). We give flowers to tell people they matter. The gift received in hospital makes fighting to get well a more attractive option, knowing that someone cares that you do. But when red roses are given, the message is more explicit. It does not communicate I care what happens, it means I am in love with you. So what does knowing someone has such deep feelings for you do to a person, I wonder.

Often there is a smile. Thoughts, perhaps, of a romance together or maybe even kids? The symbolism of the rose is timeless....it conveys the message "I'd like to feel this way about you until the end of time".

In the same way, how appropriate would it be to give red roses as a get well gift to someone *else's* wife? Or actually, to your gran? Immediately, it seems to jar. It is something that just isn't done. It is a primordial symbolism that strikes right to the core.

So, *when* we receive those red roses, from someone we adore, it *should* be that our heart soars, we hold hands and it's happily ever after. But sadly life just ain't like that, is it? The human condition unfailingly makes it harder.

Unaware of the baggage we carry from past relationships with lovers, parents and others, the hurts of our previous selves influence our emotional and physical reactions. We emotionally withhold. We are suspicious and distrusting. For many those first few nights of sex are a conflagration of passion, but sooner or later a fire extinguisher switches on and alarm bells start to ring. Tragically not all pregnancy tests turn blue and that dream of family bliss remains elusive. Even the happiest marriages have an expiry date when one lonely lover stands at a grave still unable to say goodbye. Love continues but the pain endlessly screams on.

"Where is happily ever after?" we wonder, as the fairy tale lie begins to unfurl.

But the strange and enchanting thing is the petals from that rose hold medicines incomprehensible in their power. They heal grief. Repair marriages. Unlock and dissipate trauma. Revive sexuality. Reduce anxiety. Dispel sadness. They restore trust.

Whilst *I* have written this book, it is the wisdom of other realms you find on the page. Of Ancient Sumerian Goddesses, of Cleopatra and the Early Church. Of Ayurvedic and Traditional Chinese Medicine and the extraordinary insights of the healers from so very long ago. Of modern day medicine, of nurses and midwives, addiction counsellors, doctors and scientists from across the globe. Evidential explanations of why the rose can so magically repair problems of love, grief and sex.

Truly, with this book, I am but a vessel whose fingers pitter-pattered on the keyboard...nothing more.

And yet...I am astounded by the things I have come to learn.

Whoever "they" are, they say "Listen to your intuition". I try to do that. Other people say "stick to the plan, don't get distracted and drift off on a tangent". I try to do that too. Hell, I am one of the people who say it!

And yet Rose drew me in.

It wasn't on my radar to research. Arrogantly I believed that after over twenty years of using the oil, I pretty much knew everything there was to know. And yet, people kept asking me to take a look. Robert Tisserand asked me to write a piece on rose, then Gergley Hollandi from the Hungarian aromatherapy magazine Aromatika.hu, and then the International Federation of Aromatherapists asked me, too.

Like a siren's call the fragranced magic drew me in, irresistible to ignore.

"They" also say when you are in the right place information just flows and serendipity smiles. Well serendipity was over the moon to see me turn up to her party and for three months I have had inspiration, wisdom and rose data rushing at me like a tidal wave ready to break.

The question is though...where does one start? Which is the most important aspect of the rose? Is it the laboratory trials confirming her power? Possibly. But how can one fully understand her alchemy unless the sorcery of the feminine divine is considered too?

Where does the fragrance of the rose smell strongest? Wafting from the sails of Cleopatra's gilded barge, or in the bedrooms of men rejoicing to have their sexuality returned to them? Is it concealed behind a hospital screen where nursing new mums are helped to bond with their child or in student dorms where girls are learning to better manage their menstrual pain?

Perhaps it lingers, still, in those first Islamic distilleries, or maybe in Bulgarian rose fields at dawn, where the pickers rush to gather blooms before the morning sun has chance to steal the precious scent.

Come with me, and I'll show you where happily ever after lives.

Just for a couple of hours let's escape our humdrum lives. Let's cast aside our wearied outlook, tainted by sadness and heartache and let's look at life through rose coloured glasses. We'll steal away to hillsides of pink blooms smiling beneath the rosy dawn sky. Let's immerse ourselves in the perfume secrets of the Romans and the mysterious medicines of Greece. Marvel at the spectacle of Mark Anthony's first meeting with his queen and share in her delight as her magic begins to take hold.

Peer over the shoulders of modern day lab researchers, drug counsellors and doctors alike. Read their charts with glee. Listen and you will hear a primordial whisper echoing along university corridors across the world "Didn't we tell you so? ..." seems to be the goddess sigh.

Myths and mysteries, magic and medicine...with rose all four are quintessentially the same. And when, at the end of your time machine journey across five thousand years, you place those rose coloured specs aside, I suspect that you may find you feel as I do...

That happily ever after is to be found with the petals of the rose.

Table of Contents

Chapter 1 The Rose of Antiquity

It seems to me to be a strange contradiction that the history of the rose, when her *bloom* is so ephemeral and fleeting. Her beautiful scent and extraordinary properties have a timeless grace that has *always* guaranteed her superstar status. There is fossilised evidence of wild roses growing as early as 60-70 million years ago, always north of the equator, even as far as Norway and Alaska but we have to wait many millions of years before we start to see how she became part of the symbolism, medicine and romance that we know her for today.

Perhaps her most famous connection is with Cleopatra but in fact her usage can be traced back almost three thousand years before that in its associations with the Sumerian goddess Innana. She was the paramount goddess of the Sumerian pantheon and the most loved of all the deities. She was goddess of procreation, of love and of war. The very height of her power is thought to have been around 2900BC. Innana's temple was at Uruk, not far from the bank of the Euphrates in modern day Iraq. The earliest symbol we see depicting her is reeds tied together with streamers, but later by the Sargonic period (2700-2350BC) we see her almost always depicted by an eight pointed star or a primitive picture of a rose.

Although Innana was not a mother goddess she shares many connections with other nature goddesses who were to arise in her wake in the centuries to come, most notably in terms of rose symbolism with Ishtar, Aphrodite, Venus and Isis.

A door seal dating from c3300BC was recovered in North Mesopotamia depicting two scorpions guarding the rosette of Innana which here, looks very much like an eight pointed star. It was probably meant to protect a door to a room full of offerings for the goddess and is the earliest pictorial representation we have of the flower.

The earliest written references where we hear roses actually *growing,* is found in an extraordinary archaeological haul dating from the 7th Century BC. The Royal Library of Ashurbanipal at Nineveh (again in modern day Iraq), is named after King Ashurbanipal who was the last great king of the Neo-Assyrian empire. Sadly, very little remains of the clay tablets, but the words "amurdinnu" or "murdimu" are discernible which have been translated as *Bramble Rose* or *Wild Rose.*

It seems likely then that the rose began its "career" in Persia, found its way through to Greece, and then, through Roman trade, began to emerge in Egypt around about the 6-7th century BC. The prominent American mythologist Joseph Campbell (He, who originated the mantra: "Follow your bliss",) speaks of how there are very strong parallels between the myths of Inanna, Ishtar and Isis, (indeed when the temple of Uruk was excavated in 1849 there were signs that the temple had later been dedicated to the goddess Ishtar.)

- Each of the consorts of Innana, Isis, Venus and Aphrodite is associated with the cycles of vegetation.

- All were entitled **Queen of Heaven**.

- Each represented the **cycle of love, loss, death and eventual restoration.**

- In each pantheon we see **The Queen of Heaven aligned with the rose.**

It seems fairly certain that, as the worship of the feminine divine travelled through time, across distance and through nations, so the importance of the rose travelled with her.

Excavations of Brexiza, in Attika, Southern Greece were to attest to the prominence of how Isis, consort of Osiris, God Of The Underworld, was to gain power throughout Greece. Work is still underway to preserve the Temple of Isis, today, where enormous statues of the goddess have been found. Since the original discovery of two marble statues in 1967, there have been discoveries of sphinxes and a striking statue of Isis and there she holds, of course, a rose in each of her hands.

Certainly by the height of Ancient Egyptian dominion, the rose had taken on a very clear representation.

- Full bloom represented life
- Withered bloom meant death.

This symbolism was important when laying the dead into their tombs. The rose, of course had become synonymous with Isis and "Wreaths of justification" were made for the righteous dead as a sign that the deceased had successfully passed through to the judgment hall of Osiris. Depictions of roses are found on the walls of the tomb Tutmoses VI (C14th BC). In 1888, Sir Flinders Petrie discovered garlands from a funeral wreath whilst excavating tombs in Upper Egypt. Later identified as *Rosa x richardii*, or is now known as *St John's Rose*, the desiccated petals had maintained their pinkish hue. When soaked in water they returned to near life like state.

A fascinating document is housed in the Ashmoleon Museum in Oxford, England. **The Oxyrhynchus Papyri LII 3694** was found when two young fellows from Queen's College Oxford began, half heartedly, to excavate what was, to all intents and purposes, a rubbish tip just outside the city of Oxyrhynchus. Their interest was very quickly piqued when they discovered arid conditions had preserved what was to be an extraordinary insight into life in the area, all those thousands of years before. Hundreds upon hundreds of scrap papyri, which had been written on both sides to save money, had been dumped in a heap. All manner of ancient data had been discarded here, Receipts', letters, shopping lists, business ledgers, medical texts to name but a few. It is in this ancient archive that we find reference to the Hellenic - Isis Festival of Roses, ***the Rhodophoria. The papyrus reads:***

"Invitation to strategus

To Aurelius Harpocration, strategus.

From the inhabitants and notables of the village of Serpis

The Great god Ammon, who loves you, invites you on the 16th of the present month, phaemonth, on the occasion of a festival and a rhodophoria"

Rhod / Rhodo is from the Greek word *rhodon* meaning rose

Phore/ Phorus/ Pherein – To carry/ To bear / The bearer

As yet, it is not clear what exactly happened at this event, apart from the actual carrying of roses in celebration of Isis! Some sources suggest it may be an alternative name for the spring / summer celebration called the Rosalia. This had originated as a festival to honour the dead placing flowers onto burial sites then over time had developed into a way of honouring military heroes by laying wreaths upon statues and monuments. Flowers chosen for the Rosalia were synonymous with the cycle of life: birth, life, death rebirth and these flowers framed the Rosalia season. Traditionally beginning in May, celebrations would be sprinkled through to July, the violets marking the first flower of spring and the roses, the last to bloom in the summer. The colours of the roses and violets seemed to echo the colour of blood which had been spilt and were used as a method of pleasing and appeasing their deities.

The relationship that the Egyptians had with scent is very different to ours today and it is important to gain some insights into this to be able to comprehend just how powerful the rose was to come to be. The Ancient Egyptians believed beautiful scents emanated from their deities and so, when they inhaled a fragrance, such as kyphi, their temple incense, then they entered in communication with a certain god. Rose was the flower, thus the exuding fragrance of Isis, and kyphi recipes that include rose would have been for the summoning of the goddess. .

When Cleopatra VII resolved to restore the Ptolomeic dynasty to greatness, she set about making a strategic play for Mark Anthony. This was to be one of the most dramatic seductions history had ever seen. Hollywood would have us believe that she pursued him for love but it is likely that played very little part in the matter. Sex was high on the agenda but a whole lot more was at stake than pleasure…she was executing a very deliberate and spectacular power play. This was a time in history when sex sealed political alliances of the highest order. Bedding the Roman would have been vital to her plan.

At the height of her career in 46 BC Egypt *should* have had it all. It had mineral wealth and agricultural ability to grow grain but the country was suffering famine and it was struggling. Just as Cleopatra had gained her throne through Caesar (and *her father* had also owed his throne to Roman help) she was eager to build on her Roman career position and restore the Ptolomeic dynasty to the greatness it had once enjoyed. To suggest that Cleopatra was an early spin doctor is an understatement to say the least! It is important to remember that she was *Greek*, not Egyptian, but nevertheless Cleopatra had been successful in winning the hearts of her country. Appealing to her domestic constituents by learning to speak Egyptian and adopting their cultural practices, not least their religious fervour for Isis, Cleopatra had the devoted love of her people.

In her book **Cleopatra the Great, the Woman behind the Legend** Professor Joann Fletcher describes the great queen as: *"Very much the performer, staging spectacular events to emphasise a divinity she had had since birth, Cleopatra literally transformed herself into a goddess for every occasion. Adapting her image to appeal to audiences at home and abroad she appeared as Venus in the heart of Rome, sailed across the Mediterranean as Aphrodite and restored Egypt's former empire as Isis, having absorbed all the attributes of the feminine divine."*

When she met Mark Anthony for the first time in Tarsus, in 41BC, wooing him was a political power play to ensure her success as a career pharaoh. Rumours were sent out across the kingdoms and whispers excitedly hummed of how Venus was to dine with Bacchus (which was how Mark Anthony had started to refer to himself).

Cleopatra pulled out all the stops. A delicate game of diplomacy began, with give and take of immeasurable proportions. Cleopatra furnished Mark Anthony with funds for his campaign (which would have been an immense gamble given Egypt's already shaky situation) and in return she asked for the head of her sister Arsinoe, the pretender to the Ptolemy crown. Sexual transactions for political ends are well documented for the period and whilst they became lovers at Tarsus, there is little evidence that they were *in* love. Neither statues of the period or Cleopatra's coinage show her to be the mesmeric beauty we hear of in legend, but nevertheless it would have been extremely difficult to ignore the great queen's wiles, I think.

Plutarch, a first century historian described their first meeting when he wrote of the life of Mark Anthony. We hear how her extraordinary boat wafted fragranced oils from its sails, to draw onlookers closer to the goddess. He relates:

She had faith in her own attractions, which, having formerly recommended her to Caesar and the young Pompey, she did not doubt might prove yet more successful with Antony. Their acquaintance was with her when a girl, young, and ignorant of the world, but she was to meet Antony in the time of life when women's beauty is most splendid, and their intellects are in full maturity. She made great preparations for her journey, of money, gifts, and ornaments of value, such as so wealthy a kingdom might afford, but she brought with her her surest hopes in her own magic arts and charms.

...she came sailing up the river Cydnus in a barge with gilded stern and outspread sails of purple, while oars of silver beat time to the music of flutes and fifes and harps. She herself lay all along, under a canopy of cloth of gold, dressed as Venus in a picture, and beautiful young boys, like painted Cupids, stood on each side to fan her. Her maids were dressed like Sea Nymphs and Graces, some steering at the rudder, some working at the ropes.

...perfumes diffused themselves from the vessel to the shore, which was covered with multitudes, part following the galley up the river on either bank, part running out of the city to see the sight. The market place was quite emptied, and Antony at last was left alone sitting upon the tribunal; while the word went through all the multitude, that Venus was come to feast with Bacchus for the common good of Asia.

On her arrival, Antony sent to invite her to supper. She thought it fitter he should come to her; so, willing to show his good humor and courtesy, he complied, and went. He found the preparations to receive him magnificent beyond expression, but nothing so admirable as the great number of lights; for on a sudden there was let down altogether so great a number of branches with lights in them so ingeniously disposed, some in squares, and some in circles, that the whole thing was a spectacle that has seldom been equalled for beauty.

Whilst we have no documentation to confirm exactly what the perfumes wafting from the sails were, common opinions seem to agree that they were probably rose and neroli oils. Certainly later in their visit, rose becomes one of the stars of history's greatest show.

The following passage is taken from a translation of *Deipnosophistae by Athenaeus* which dates from the third century AD.

Socrates of Rhodes, in the third book of the Civil War, describes the banquet given by Cleopatra, the last queen of Egypt, who married the Roman general, Antony, in Cilicia. His words are: "Meeting Antony in Cilicia, Cleopatra arranged in his honour a royal symposium, in which the service was entirely of gold and jewelled vessels made with exquisite art; even the walls, says Socrates, were hung with tapestries made of purple and gold threads. And having spread twelve triclinia, Cleopatra invited Antony and his chosen friends. He was overwhelmed with the richness of the display; but she quietly smiled and said that all these things were a present for him; she also invited him to come and dine with her again on the morrow, with his friends and his officers. On this occasion she provided an even more sumptuous symposium by far, so that she caused the vessels which had been used on the first occasion to appear paltry; and once more she presented him with these also. As for the officers, each was allowed to take away the couch on which he had reclined; even the sideboards, as well as the spreads for the couches, were divided among them. And when they departed, she furnished litters for the guests of high rank, with bearers, while for the greater number she provided horses gaily caparisoned with silver-plated harness, and for all she sent along Ethiopian slaves to carry the torches. On the fourth day she distributed fees, amounting to a talent, for the purchase of roses, and the floors of the dining-rooms were strewn with them to the depth of a cubit, in net-like festoons spread over all."

So measurements then:

How big was a cubit? Well, it depended on the length of your arm, but somewhere between 17-21 inches.

And how much was a talent? Sources suggest a **talent** typically weighed about 33 kg (75 lb) and might vary from 20 to 40 kg. Currently the international **price** of gold is about US$600 per troy ounce so one gram **costs** about $20. At this price then, a **talent** (33 kg) would be **worth** about $660,000.

So they were a foot and a half deep in roses costing well over half a million dollars! I'd have been impressed. Wouldn't you?

It's worth taking a step back here, because it is very easy to get carried away and to imagine that the queen drenched herself in the rose oil that we recognise today. But historically that cannot be so. Distillation had not yet been discovered and would not be for at least another nine hundred years.

For the most part, the rose oil of the ancient Egyptians was a product we know as **Rhodhion.** This following section is taken from Lise Manniche's book *Sacred Luxuries; Fragrance, Aromatherapy and Cosmetics of Ancient Egypt*. Many of you will have read it before in my Complete Guide, but it bears repetition, here, I think.

Rhodhion (Dioscorides)

- Oil 9.220kg
- 1000 rose petals
- Camel grass
- 2.494 kg aspalathos
- (sweet flag)
- Honey
- Salt
- Alkanet

"Bruise the camel grass, macerate with water, boil it stirring it up and down" and strain it into the oil. Throw in the "not wet" rose petals (i.e. free from dew), and, with your hands, anointed in honey, stir them "up and down" squeezing them gently every now and then. Leave them over night, and then squeeze them out. Cast the strained roses into the labellum vessel, pour 3.772 kg of the thickened oil upon them. Strain again. Pour more oil unto the roses and strain again. This will be your second oil. You may repeat this a third and fourth time

(to make a third and fourth oil), but you will anoint the vessel with honey each time. If you want to make a second transfusion (of each of these four oils) proceed with fresh dew free roses up until seven times, but no further. Always anoint your hands and the vessel with honey, stir up and down, and make sure that no juice is left with the oil, or else it will corrupt it."

She also cites a very wise prescription from a Coptic text of a treatment for the anus using rose:

"vitriol of copper; onion leaves, roasted euphorbia, leaves of marshmallow. Pound it together with oil of roses" Then the astute and clearly seasoned physician suggests that it is applied using an ibis feather, then drily comments "But first claim your fee!" Heavens above, I should say so!

Later she describes of Pliny suggests chicory used with rose oil and vinegar is the advised treatment to relieve a headache.

Sick testicles received rose action too, according to another Coptic papyrus. *"Take yellow sweet clover, rose and bride's wreath. These should be ground together and drunk with wine.*" The author then solemnly declares "With the help of God he will recover".

Theophrastus, a Greek philosopher and successor to Aristotle lived between 371-c287 BC and wrote a number of treatises on plants. One particular work, "**Concerning Odours**" is particularly illuminating about how plants were used during this period. Since the translation is now out of copyright, I can be generous with Theophastrus's wit and intellect.

The translation is a superlative piece of literature which is easy for even the most lay-person to feel Egypt and Greece come to life. I can only see one issue that might cause you real difficulties and that is ***kyphos***, a reference that appears time and again in Theophastrus's writings. In his book the Geographical Distribution of Animals and Plants Vol 2, C. Pickering suggests that kyphos may be referring to henna. He describes how Pliny and Dioscordes discuss the usage of a plant "the bruised leaves of which redden the hair) this argument carries more weight since the discoveries of mummies with their nails henna'd. Also *Megaleion* is mentioned often which is a perfume of Greek origin made from cinnamon, myrrh and charred frankincense.

- *Sesame-oil however receives rose-perfume better than other oils because of its viscid quantity; and, when subjected to fire, it gives out a smell of sesame, as though it were being disintegrated.*

- *Into rose-perfume moreover is put a quantity of salt: this treatment is peculiar to that perfume, and involves a great deal of waste, twenty-three gallons of salt being put to eight gallons and a half of the perfume.*

Perfumes are compounded from various parts of the plant, flowers leaves twigs root wood fruit and gum: and in most cases the perfume is made from a mixture of several parts. Rose and gilliflower perfumes are made from the flowers:

Some perfumes are made up colourless, some are given a colour. They give a colour to sweet marjoram-perfume, rose-perfume, and megaleion, while among expensive kinds the Egyptian, quince-perfume and kypros are colourless, as well as all the cheaper kinds. The reason why these are made without colour is that it is desired that the Egyptian and kypros should look white and that quince-perfume should have the colour of quinces, while it is not worthwhile to add colour to the cheaper sorts. The dye used for colouring red perfumes is alkanet; the sweet marjoram-perfume is dyed with the substance called khroma (dye), which is a root imported from Syria.

Medicinal uses for rose perfume:

Megaleion is believed to relieve the inflammation caused by any wound, and rose-perfume to be excellent for the ears. And this is probable enough. For the former is composed, as was said, of burnt resin cassia cinnamon and myrrh, and all these have astringent and drying properties: while the reason why rose-perfume is good for the ears is that salt is used in the manufacture of it: for it is by reason of the salt that it dries and warms (which is why 'sea-foam is also good for the ears).

Properties of certain perfumes:

The lightest are rose-perfume and kypros, which seem to be the best suited to men, as also is lily-perfume. The best for women are myrrh-oil, megaleion, the Egyptian, sweet marjoram, and spikenard: for these owing to their strength and substantial character do not easily evaporate and are not easily made to disperse, and a lasting perfume is what women require.

If one has regard to the virtues of the perfumes in question, one may well be surprised at what happens in the case of rose-perfume: – though it is lighter and less powerful than any other, if one has first been scented with it, it destroys the odour of the others. And this is why perfumers, if a purchaser hesitates and is not inclined to buy this perfume, scent him with it so that he is not able to smell the others. The explanation is that, being very delicate and acceptable to the sense of smell, by reason of its lightness it penetrates as no other can and fills up the passages of the sense, so that being entirely taken up and filled with it, it is unable to judge of others.

It is also thought that the rose even weakens the effect of compound perfume; for, when the flower is at its best, they treat compound perfumes with it; and, when these come to be opened, they smell only or chiefly of rose. However this effect is only temporary and transient because of the weakness and delicacy of the rose-scent, (the very quality which also causes it to assert itself over the scent of the other ingredients). For, as it is so delicate and is compressed by confinement, it is exhaled before the others and disperses in all directions. It is also for this reason that the rose-scent only asserts itself for a short time and then is overpowered again; for anything that is delicate and subtle must be lacking in vigour.

The reason for this is plain in view of what has been already said, seeing that this perfume overpowers others and penetrates everywhere. For the others that are heady are heavy because they are made of heavy substances, whether roots or juices; while this perfume is both light as to its scent and also by its heat well adapted to bring the passages to a suitable temperature and to open them.

And for all such purposes heat is useful, both for removing the moisture or air, and, still more, for raising the temperature of the passages and opening them: and to these ends it is helpful that the perfume should have been prepared with salt, since the effect of salt is to open the passages and to warm them thoroughly. Again the fragrance also supplies a stimulus to movement.

This perfume is also considered to be good against lassitude, because its heat and its lightness make it suitable, and also because it penetrates to the inner passages. Some however say that kypros is quite as effectual: for this too has a delicate scent which is grateful to the skin. These and similar properties may be considered peculiar to these particular perfumes.

Over time, worship of Isis becomes ever more a part of Greek culture, and reverence to rose does too. Aphrodite and the Roman Venus both also start to wear the rose mantle. Soon we also begin to see the birth of a new religion entirely, that of Christianity. Now the symbolism of the rose begins to change and take on a whole new innocent slant as the church starts to take ownership of the flower.

(It is worth commenting here, I think, that the rose does not appear in the Bible. There is reference to The Rose of Sharon, but more recent research has shown this was most probably an etiological error in translation. Nowadays, it is widely accepted that the Rose of Sharon was *Narcissus minuta,* a teeny tiny daffodil. Also Rose of Jericho appears and again...not a member of the rose family but a resurrection plant *Anastatica hierochuntica* that revives itself after years of drought on receiving a drink of water. A most unsightly specimen and un-rose like in the extreme!)

The Romans were passionate in their adoration of roses but grew them mainly in the Middle East. It is recorded that at the fall of the Roman Empire in AD 476, there were no less than 2000 public rose gardens. Cleopatra most certainly knew her target audience well, because to a Roman a rose was something very special, their love of the flower bordering on obsession. They were strewn at public ceremonies and banquets. The Emperors fountains spurted gallons of rosewater and public baths were filled with the same. Awnings in amphitheatres were steeped in rose oil so that the sun released a godlike scent as they sat in repose. Legend has it that the Emperor Nero was so smitten with rose that he had silver pipes installed beneath plates at the banquet table of his Roman orgy, the Bachurnalia. Rosewater spritzed them as they relaxed between courses. A celestial rose mural was painted onto the ceiling above them, and petals cascaded down upon his guests. On one occasion, so many fell, it is told, one diner was inadvertently smothered to death!

Pillows were stuffed with them, beautiful ointments and sprays were concocted and delicious custards were all made with petals.

It is likely that this obsession with the flower is the reason for the later references to the Madonna (and on occasion the Christ Child) as The Rose. Roman followers of Christ, at the time, were well known for taking versions of Egyptian and Greek religions and integrating them into church practices (Sunday as the Sabbath was for convenience of worshippers of the sun god Ra). Taking the rose as a symbol of the virgin was an easy way to erase Isis/ Aphrodite and Venus from the pagan ways. In the church, doctrine was to follow "Thou shalt worship no other God but me." The days of polytheistic worship were over. The goddesses they let go, with relative ease, but the rose…well, it seemed she had to stay.

Clearly though, where she had previously been the embodiment of procreation of delicious and voluptuous sexual liaison, over time she was to become a far paler shade of herself. A white rose often replacing the red.

I think it is interesting to look at how the rose is depicted in early Christianity in this period too. In the eyes of the puritanical early church the flower, with its associations with paganistic rituals, naturally became associated with orgies and of salacious lust. In AD 202 one of the foremost Christian authors wrote a huge work outlawing roses and forbidding them to grow, or for people to have them in their houses. Presumably then these many Roman rose gardens belonged to non-Christians of the period.

Over the succeeding years it became clear that in order to strengthen the attractiveness of the church, they would have to absorb some of the pagan doctrine and gradually roses became part of their theology. It is not uncommon in hymns and oratorios for the Virgin Mary to be referred to "Rosa Mystica" or "the Rose without thorns".

After the fall of Rome, Europe struggled with various battles and wars and it became virtually impossible to maintain their belovèd formal rose gardens in the same way. This structured fashion of gardens went into decline and faded into history.

Really, we must thanks monks for preserving plant medicine through this time. Potentially the only thing that saved roses from being wiped out was the fact that monasteries had to have just one rose plant so a chosen scholar could study its medicinal properties.

Crusaders returned to Europe in the 12th century regaling tales of wonderful roses they had found in the Middle East. They, of course, brought sample plants and resurrected Europe's deep love for gardens.

From here then, we need to step back into our rose scented Tardis in order to fill in some of the blanks that had arisen in different parts of the world. Whilst Europe was entering The Dark Ages and the rose was suffering its decline, the Arabs were making busy indeed, inventing all manner of processes and equipment, not least those we now know as distillation.

Chapter 2 Unani Medicine's Gift of Rose

It is undecided where the original rose essence, as we know it today originated. We have evidence of rose*water* being distilled as early as the 9th century. It seems fairly likely that the essential oil was a lucky accident arising from this. Two cultures claim responsibility for this.

Abu Yusuf Yakub Ishak Al Kindi was a 9th Century Arab philosopher, born and educated in, what we would call, modern day Basra in Iraq. Studying in Baghdad, he became well versed in the writings of Aristotle. Often referred to as the Philosopher of The Arabs, he is recognised as the earliest of the philosophers of Muslim descent.

Al Kindi wrote *Kitab Kimya' Al 'Itr wa Al Tas'idat* , **The Book of Distillation and Chemistry**. Here we find early explanations of how essences could be extracted from host plants. Besides his writings on philosophy he produced over 250 treatises on a variety of subjects. Sadly, only a few concerning medicine and astrology are now still in existence.

Detailing descriptions of distillation methods for 107 species of plants The Book of Distillation and Chemistry encompasses an epic 71 chapters. Each plant, he relates, requires slightly different concerns and methods of care to obtain their valuable elixir.

Later, a pre-eminent medieval Muslim surgeon *Abulcasis* describes in his work **"In Pharmacy**" how he has seen vinegar being distilled "**in a container very similar to that used to contain rosewater**"

So we know for sure that ***rosewater*** was in existence and was being produced at least in the 10th Century. It is not until 17th century Indian writings, however that we catch a glimpse of the **rose attar** we know today. It is likely that wisdom of medicinal properties of rose travelled with the knowledge of an ancient medical system called Unani.

Practiced across the Arabic world, Hindustan and Pakistan, Unani is, today, the traditional medicine of Southern Asia. Originally a Greco-Arabic medicine derived from the same roots as western medicine, (that is from the teachings of Hippocrates and Galen) it gained a great deal of popularity in the Middle Ages.

Considered to date back to about 1025AD it is thought that Unani medicine arrived in India in or around the 12th or 13th Centuries AD.

Unani encompasses a wide range of practices including Turkish baths, cupping, promotion of sweating and diuretics, purging and emetics of detoxification and massage. It is here too, that we first really see aromatherapy as an art discussed explicitly in ancient medical texts. Here it referred to as a mechanism of action that stimulates the olfactory nerve and subsequently the brain

Primarily based upon Greek and Arabic medicines, it also drew on the Sushrata and Charaka Samhitas, the ancient texts which form the basis of Ayurveda. It is at this time that we see the coming together of many different disciplines that were to bring rose to the very forefront of cultural melting pot of medicines.

Much of the knowledge of Unani medicine comes from the writings of Avicenna, a scholar and physician from the early 10th Century. His most famous works are *The Book of Healing* which is a philosophical and scientific work and *The Canon of Medicine* – which forms a very early medical encyclopaedia. The Canon of Medicine later became a standard medical text for study in medieval universities. His work remained in use as late as 1650.

Medieval wisdom from Avicenna and His Canon of Medicine

The very first lesson I took in aromatherapy was about the history of aromatherapy and it spoke of Avicenna (which is the Romanised version of his real name Ali Abu Ibn Sena) I have to confess, though I never knew very much more about him than his name. It was fascinating, then, for me to scour a translation of his ***Canon of Medicine.***

He describes the spirit thus:

"fluid believed to act as a medium between mind and the grosser matter of the body."

" a kind of very subtle body which penetrates all parts of the material body and infuses them like the essence of a rose, oil in sesame, butter in milk"

Here are some of his prescriptions describing how rosewater was used at the end of the first millennium. I think you'll particularly enjoy his notes on bathing!

Shower-baths, Douching, Spraying. –

If water be sprinkled on the face (or over the body) it restores the vigour of the breath, when that has been lost by dyspnoea and by the inflammatory changes in hot fevers. .This sprinkling is especially beneficial for syncope, if rose water or vinegar be used. It may restore the appetite. They are injurious to persons suffering from catarrhs or "cold" headaches.

Digestive Problems

"Modern teaching: Vomiting and diarrhoea must always be looked upon as due to some cause other than dentition, particularly to improper feeding – If it is only slight, you will not be asked to treat it. If the parents are afraid it will become injurious, leading to wasting, one would treat by applying rose-seed, caraway, anise, and celery (parsley-) seed [sprinkled on wool : Aeg.] to the abdomen, or apply a plaster prepared with caraway and roses infused in vinegar, or with frumenty boiled in, vinegar.

Digestive disturbance/ Weakness of the stomach.

The abdomen should be anointed with musk and rose or myrtle water. Give a drink containing quince juice and a little clove or nutmeg, or three-eighths of a dram of nutmeg with a small quantity of quince-juice.

Sunstroke

Inflammation in the brain. Siriasis (Greek translation – sunstroke).

There is pain in the eyes and the throat, and the face becomes yellow. [The body is dry; the fontanelles are depressed, the orbits sunken

Hence the brain must be rendered cool and moist by the use of cortex of cucumber, parings of gourd, juice of garden nightshade, and especially purslane juice, and rose oil with a little vinegar, and rose oil with egg-yolk. Each of these is constantly changed.

Mouth Ulcers

[The] membrane of the tongue and mouth is too delicate to bear touching, even by the wateriness of the milk, for it is this that is injurious to it, and gives rise to" the aphthae. The condition

is worse, and dangerous to life, if they remain immature and black like charcoal. The condition is more favourable if they are white or yellow. The treatment is to employ some such gentle medication as -is described in special treatises on the subject. Sometimes triturated violets are sufficient by them- selves ; sometimes they need mixing with roses, a little saffron and carob-bean. Or, again, lettuce-juice, nightshade juice, purslane juice [and endive-juice] may 'suffice. If treatment is still resisted, use bruised liquorice root.

Prolapsus ani (Rectal Prolapse)

Give pomegranate bark, fresh myrrh, inner rinds of acorns (or, chestnuts), dried roses, burnt horn' alum of Yamen, nails of goats, pomegranate blossoms (unopened) and nails of fowls. Take equal parts and thoroughly boil them ogether in water until all their virtue has come out. Then give as an enema, tepid.

Spots and Skin Problems

The treatment in all cases [of pimples on the skin] consists in using fine desiccants dissolved in the bath-water, such remedies as rose, myrtle, mastic-leaves, tamarisk, and their respective oils being boiled in the water. [Other remedies recommended by Alsaharavius :lotions of marjoram, mint, centaury ; ointments of spuma argenti, ceruse, armenian bole, sulphur, mercury, almonds.]

If they become vesicular, they should be steamed, and have water poured over them in which myrtle and rose and bogrush (schoenus), quinsywort- (asperula) and the (young) leaves of the mastic tree have been boiled.

For vesicular eruptions, Rhazes advises : (i) decoction of dates and figs with fennel-water ; (2) when the rash is fully out, give rose-water baths, myrtle-water baths, and then rub the skin with oil of roses.

Intertrigo. Apply ground myrtle as a dusting powder, or use powdered liquorice root [or iris root] ; or finely ground-up rose or galangale, or barley flour, or lentil flour.

Bathing

Friction. Massage. Shampooing

"Abu Sir came to him and rubbed his body with the bag-gloves, peeling from his skin dirt-rolls like lamp-wick, and showing them to the King, who rejoiced therein . . . after which thorough washing, Abu Sir mingled rose-water with the water of the tank, and the King went down therein. When he came

forth his body was refreshed, and he felt a lightness and liveliness such as he had never known m his life."

Bad Temper

(Because of its affects on the liver and bile)

Where there is any risk of the bilious humour undergoing fermentative decomposition, and one wishes to bathe fasting, the aliment should be attenuant. But a person of hot temperament' in whom the bilious humour is plentiful, should not enter the hot chamber at all. The best things for such persons to take are: bread soaked with the juice of fruits or rose-water.

Over Eating

When a -state of over-repletion exists in regard to some meal, whether as a result of exercise (which causes undue hunger), or because a draught has been taken as well, then there will be a need for rapid emesis. If this should fail, or one cannot vomit, .the person should sip hot water until the repletion is displaced and sleep supervenes. The person should therefore lie down and (compose himself to) sleep. Let him sleep as long as he will. – But should this not suffice, or should he be unable to go to sleep, . ; reflect whether the natural course of events is likely to save you from procuring emesis. If so, good. If not, assist the natural power by any gentle laxative, such as myrobalan electuary, confection of roses, or origanum prepared with sugar or honey ; or by the use of such things as cumin, spiced candies, asphodel and cabbage ptisan.

It was very interesting for me to see a report emerge, whilst I was writing this section, about a translation, completed this month by Greek scholars, of a very ancient manuscript dating from the 13th Century. The document is a detailed analysis of plants used as antidotes used in the Byzantine Empire. The writings, which form the first chapter of a far bigger work known as Element Alpha by Nicolas Myrepsos, recount antidotal properties of 39 medicinal plants. The Apiacea genus, which contains plants such as celery, carrot and parsley, seems to frequent the most often at just over 10% of the instances. Rose features about half as often but in all cases it is R*osa centifolia* that is cited, not The Damask Rose. You can find details of the work here: http://www.ncbi.nlm.nih.gov/pubmed/?term=Nikolaos+Myrepsos

It is interesting, I think, to just run a cursory glance over the basics of unani medicine to be able to understand how it sits within the Eastern Medicines.

You will recall that Ayurveda works on a three dosha system, that of vata, pitta, kapha. By contrast Traditional Chinese Medicine (TCM) works on a five element system that of Earth, Air, Fire Water and Ether. Unani sits in between using four elements which we describe as humours. Just as we see properties in the doshas, such as vata as being dry and cool, and pitta being hot and moist, so Unani has its own similar descriptors.

These are:

- **Balgham - Phlegm - Cold/wet**
- **Dam - Blood - Hot/Wet**
- **Safra -Yellow Bile - Hot/ Dry**
- **Sanda - Black Bile - Cold/dry**

The premise of this medicine is that disease is a natural process and that symptoms are nothing more than the body's natural reaction to disease. Here then we see a similar ideal of an ongoing preventative medicine, just as in Ayurveda, rather than plants being viewed as a cure.

The Unani name of *Rosa damascena* is **Roghan-e Gul.** It is advertised for sale by the same name today.

Here we find it used for:

- Mouth ulcers – petals mixed with borax and made into a poultice
- Thrush, (unclear whether it is oral or vaginal but I think the former) - petals mixed with borax and made into a poultice
- Early stages of meningitis - petals soaked into sesame oil and rubbed onto the forehead and then covered with a vinegar soaked flannel and ice
- Heat headaches
- Delirium caused by fever
- Insomnia

Traditional usage of rose in Unani medicine seems to have been:

- Chest and abdominal pain
- Strengthening the heart
- Digestive
- Menstrual problems

- Inflammation- especially of the neck

It is seen to be

- Anti HIV
- Antibacterial
- Anti tussive (stops you coughing)
- Hypnotic
- Anti diabetic

The word attar comes from the Arabic word *'itr* which was to travel with the essence thus far to its existence today.

In his memoirs, the 17th-century Mughal emperor Jahangir speaks of how his mother-in-law, Salima Sultan Begum was to uncover Attar of Roses entirely by chance.

"This 'itr is a discovery which was made during my reign by the mother of Nur Jahan Begum." He continues "When she was making rose water, a scum formed on the surface of the dishes into which the hot rose water was poured from the jugs.

She collected this scum little by little; when much rose water was obtained a considerable quantity of the scum was collected."

It becomes very clear here that the Emperor did, indeed have an intimate acquaintance of the magical elixir that had been brought forth as he describes perfectly the aromatherapy properties we use today.

He relates: ***"It is of such strength in perfume that if one drop be rubbed on the palm of the hand it scents a whole assembly and it seems as if many red rosebuds had bloomed at once. There is no other scent of equal excellence to it. It restores hearts that have gone and brings back withered souls. In reward for that invention, I presented a string of pearls to the inventor. Salima Sultan Begum—may the light of God be upon her tomb—gave this oil the name 'itr-i-Jahangiri."***

Socially, even today rosewater is sprinkled at weddings to ensure a happy event. Achingly beautiful silver sprays can still be found which have been passed down many generations of family events.

In Iran, the rose is known as *Gole Mohammadi*- That is Flower of The Prophet, because the beautiful fragrance reminds them of the presence of the prophet. (How similar this is to the ideas of the Ancient Egyptians.)

In Saudi Arabia, a rose species called the Taif rose is grown, which is botanically very similar to the rose we find in Bulgaria. There, their rose is seen as a symbol of love, of purity and of meditation and prayer.

It is thought that about two centuries ago, Arabian distillers took their art to Taif to locate themselves closer to Mecca, helping them to prevent the loss of precious vapours which might escape during transit to the Holy City. Soon, after the distilleries were established in Taif, Taif Rose Oil was to become infamous across the entirety of the Muslim world.

Outside of the Sacred Mosque in Mecca, Taif rose is used in the sanctifying ritual, *Kaaba*. The washing ritual of the Kaaba begins with the performance of two raka'hs (prayers) inside of The House of God. The interior walls are then cleansed with rose, Oudh and musk perfumes. Water from the Holy Zamzam well is mixed with rose perfume, splashed onto the floor and then wiped fresh with bare hands and palm leaves.

Pilgrims coming from the East will very often take a route via Taif in the sole objective of buying some of this precious rose oil. Any Muslim able afford it will buy at least one vial of this very precious rose oil as a souvenir of Hajj.

The **Delhi Sultanate** was a period in Indian history that stretches for 320 years (from 1206-1526) and a time of great learning. Science, mathematics, philosophy and medicine all flourished. The second ruler of the Khulji Dynasty, **Alauddin Khilji**, was considered to be the most powerful of the regime. Kulji retained several eminent Unani physicians (known as Hakims) in his courts. His patronage of the art of Unani, and the great wealth of literature and practice that took place during this period ensured that the medicine grew in strength and popularity. As is the wont of any good healer, Ayurvedic practitioners were eager to discover the secrets of Western Medicine and the practices became irreversibly enmeshed. The edges become blurred and from here on in, it becomes impossible to extricate Eastern from Western medicine especially where rose is concerned.

Chapter 3 Rose – an Ayurvedic Medicine

The rose of Ayurveda is **shatapattri,** which means a hundred petals and is what we, in aromatherapy, call *Rosa centifolia.*

It coordinates the conversation between *prana vata* and balances *sadarkha pitta.*

- **Prana vata** rules the head, brain, chest and respiratory system, as well as sensory perception.
- **Sadarka pitta** is a subdosha of pitta that pertains to the emotions and their *effect on the heart.*

Prana Vata governs:

- Movement of mind, thoughts and feelings

It correlates with the neural activities of the brain

It promotes:

- Enthusiasm
- Inspiration

- Mental adaptability
- Ability to communicate
- The ability to co-ordinate ideas in the mind

Out of balance, prana vata can lead to behaviour that is:

- Anxious, disorganised, ungrounded, overwhelmed, fearful, spacey, insecure
- Wakefulness between 2-6am
- Neurological problems such as palpitations, tremors, Parkinson's, epilepsy and depression

Long term it is likely you will see a person become:

- exhausted, suffer from chronic anxiety, panic attacks, changeable but intense depression

Sadarkha pitta is said to dwell in the heart and to circulate its energy. Its properties and thus the action of rose on the spirit are:

- Decisiveness

- Desire
- Drive
- The ability to analyse and discriminate
- Intelligence
- Contentment
- Motivation
- Self confidence
- Memory
- Emotional balance
- Our ability to feel fulfilment
- And to a certain extent spirituality
- Certainly it controls our ability to fulfil our goals whether those be material or spiritual

Physically:

- It governs homeostasis

- The hypothalamus
- And the balance between the hormones

In Ayurveda the heart is said to have two energies

- Agni - solar energy
- Soma- Lunar energy

Sadarka pitta connects the heart and mind energetically so they can communicate. A channel, if you like, for information to the brain. This data encompasses ideas, impressions and thoughts, taking them from external information, to the brain and then to the heart.

This data is known as *manovaha srotas.*

How effectively manovaha srotas travels through the system relies entirely on the strength of sadarkha pitta. Consider it to be the engine driving the portal train of information, if you like.

Rose ignites agni and through this balances the action. If agni burns too brightly it will burn away soma energy and we see reduced levels of *ojas* or vitality. In some ways we can say that sadarka is like agni, in that just as agni is responsible for the internal digestive fire, sadarka pitta cooks our experiences. If the energy is too low then we cannot process either sensory or emotional input and the feelings become stagnant and impossible to come to terms with. Too strong and we have volcanic, out of proportion reactions to them.

In balance then, we are even tempered. Out of balance, it is likely that you will see anger, moodiness, irritability and sadness.

The more in excess this energy becomes you can see the person edging towards being domineering, controlling, critical (and here I mean both to themselves and of others). It becomes very hard for them to concentrate. They can often become manipulative too. (Can you see how we have this overlap with energy that we saw in the vetiver book?)

Physically, how are they sleeping? When this goes awry the chances are they will be waking up far too early all fired up for the day with their head buzzing with ideas. You are going to see inflammation too of some description, whether we think allergies, dermatitis, heartburn or diarrhoea. Predictably, if external stress or grief affects this channel we will see the heart affected on a more physical level. *Vyana vata* governs the circulation concerning pressure of both the blood and oxygen too.

So how did the person get like this? Well, Ayurveda says that sadarka pitta is aggravated by **hot weather** or **getting overheated** somehow. **Drinking excess alcohol, eating too much white sugar** and red meat will also cause difficulties. **Working or living in violent situations** will also inflame the situation too.

We have a chicken and egg situation, too, when we think of menopause and PMT, which came first, the hormone issues, the nasty temper or the ten ton of chocolate we washed down with red wine?

There is never really any new wisdom is there? Simply different translations of the same.

Rose petals are often used in Rasayanas, which I talk about quite extensively in my book about Holy Basil.

The term *Rasayana* comes from the very earliest Ayurvedic texts and its English translation from the Sanskrit means "The Science of Lengthening Life". In texts later than the 8th Century the meaning takes on a slightly different slant and it becomes the name of Indian Alchemy.

Here, tonics are made from rose paste, adding spices and water. These pastes are also often used as a salve to cool burning.

Much emphasis is placed on the consumption of rose petal spread (we saw Avicenna refer to it as rose confection) and it is said that taking 1-2 tea spoons a day will draw away feeling of suspicion and sadness. Generally, daily consumption helps a person to think more positively.

Chapter 4 The Rose & Chinese Medicine (TCM)

I have not been able to trace how recently roses found their way to China, since they seem to appear far less common in literature and art than say, the chrysanthemum. It would seem that are comparative newcomers to Chinese plants, only mentioned as far back as the 14th century BC. In truth though, no one knows how long roses have been cultivated, grown and loved in China. What is clear though is that China has enjoyed a passionate love affair with the plant for a very long time.

In 500AD Confucius writes of the many roses growing in the Imperial Gardens, and he also describes the Chinese Emperors library as housing hundreds of books about roses. The rose gardeners of the Han Dynasty (207BC-AD220) were so passionate about the flower, that the Emperor is said to have convened because the rose gardens were over whelming land which was allotted for growing provisions and food. Then, in the Chinese Floral Encyclopaedia *Zhongguo Huajing, a* widespread rose culture is described throughout the 4th and 5th centuries AD. By the Song Dynasty (960 to 1279 AD), we find references to "Yuejihua," incredible perpetual-flowering roses extensively cultivated in larger cities housing large numbers of varieties.

Unlike in Aromatherapy where we really only use two varieties of rose *Rosa damascena* and on very rare occasions *Rosa centifolia,* Traditional Chinese Medicine employs several species, all with very slightly different properties.

Mei Gui Hua - Rosa Rugosa

Young Flower of the Chinese Rose

This bud is the closest to the romantic pink roses we know and probably has the most similar effects to aromatherapy's damascena.

This rose has sweet, slightly bitter and warming properties.

- It is associated with the liver and spleen meridians.
- It regulates and promotes the movement of qi and reduces stagnation.

- It nourishes the skin
- It improves digestion
- It relieves liver and stomach disharmony that can lead to distension in the flanks.
- Belching
- Calming to the pain of mastitis (sore breasts)
- Balances the endocrine system
- Soothes the mood
- Enriches the blood and qi
- Nourishes the skin
- Eliminates fatigue
- Improves digestion
- Reduces bruising
- Invigorates poor appetite
- Harmonises the blood

- Disperses statis – this might mean circulatory or emotional stasis from trauma

Rose is used here for distended stomach, epigastric pain, pain from external injuries, and irregular menses. It stimulates the gynaecological system and it harmonises the spleen.

Yueji – Rosa Chinensis

Translation – *China Rose*

- Used for regulation of menses
- Treatment of enlarged thyroid gland

Jin Ying Zi - Rosa laevigata

Translation - Cherokee Rose

American readers may be stopped in their tracks to see that the state flower of Georgia is such an important medicine in China. The delicate white bloom with its bright yellow centre growing wild along your hedgerows is said to have gained its name as the Cherokees moved from Mississippi to Oklahoma. Following the Indian Removal Act 1830, the Cherokee Indians were forced to leave their ancestral homes and move to a designated territory just south of Mississippi. Few children survived the arduous exodus, and on hearing the wails of the grieving mothers, the elders asked for a sign to sustain them. The next day it is said that a rose blossomed on the site of every tear to fall along the "Trail of Tears".

The Cherokee rose originally came from China. Usage in Chinese Medicine is mainly of the rose hips harvested in Sept-Oct. Thorns are taken off and the seeds are removed. The hips are then left to dry in the sun.

It is astringent to the large intestine and so we also see it being the prescription of choice for diarrhoea too. Modern research shows that the diarrhoea is calmed by Cherokee rose's ability to cause a contraction of the intestinal mucosa. Because it is calming is also an excellent remedy for chronic gastroenteritis.

According to, ***Ten Lectures on the use of Medicinals from the personal experience of Jiao Shu-De (Jiao Clinical Chinese Medicine*** treatment with Cherokee rose would be contraindicated when there is pain associated with urination that would indicate " an excess of repletion heat and evil fire" in the kidney.

One of the most important usages of the Cherokee rose is for *spermatorrhea*. This is a very common ailment where a male ejaculates small amounts of semen outside of intercourse. I'll cover this in more detail in a moment because this is probably the point, I think, where rose medicine becomes most fascinating! To understand this medicine, it is necessary to explore an aspect of their medicinal theory called *jing*.

The Action of Rose on Jing or

The Essence of the Body

Jing is the Chinese word for "**essence**" and more specifically *kidney* essence. It is one of the Three Treasures of TCM (the others being ***qi*** and ***shen***, whose closest translation might be spirit). It is thought that **rose strengthens the essence gate and prevents a loss of jing**.

We first see jing explained in ***Huangdi Neijing, The Yellow Emperors Classic of Internal Medicine***. This has formed the basis of Traditional Chinese Medicine for over two thousand years. The text is split into two parts and forms conversations between the mystical Emperor Huangdi and his six ministers.

The first text 素問 *Suwen* refers to Basic Questions and for the main part this pertains to diagnosis. The second part is less often referred to, lingshu 靈樞, and explains fully the practice of acupuncture. It is unknown really when the Neijing originates from, with estimations being somewhere between the Warring period (475-221 BC) and the last Han Dynasty(206 BCE–220 CE) but most commonly held belief is that is probably dates to the second century BC. It is an important work because it is the first time we see the idea that illness does not arise from demons but from internal processes affected by diet etc.

The text relates that jing is **stored within the kidneys** and it is the **densest physical matter in the body** (in contrast to shen which is deemed to be the most volatile, so I find it easiest to imagine this as if it were our western states of matter: jing being thick liquid as opposed to the gaseous, more ethereal state of shen).

Jing governs the material basis of the body, so: **the blood, the tissues, bones** and **teeth**. It is predominately **yin in nature.** Things that are yin, you might recall from my Vetiver and Monarda books are cooling, drying and nourishing. The biggest physical strains on jing are production of semen in men, and menstrual blood (and pregnancy too) in women. A person is born, it is said, with a *fixed* amount of jing. Post natally it is nourished by food but also exercise, study and meditation.

From the moment a child is born, jing begins to deplete. Daily illness, every day stress, substance abuse and sexual challenges begin to steal its energy. Whilst it is very difficult to ever recapture and renew the levels of jing we are born with, taking care of the levels can help to bolster and preserve it. As a child begins to breath, eat and of course, think independently of their parents, all of their systems (respiratory, digestion et al) become intricately involved in how well jing is conserved. When we finally leave this earthly realm, all jing is considered to be consumed.

Jing is thought to be passed to the foetus from the parents, and to be the carrier of our heritage (similar to

DNA, if you like). Throughout the pregnancy, jing, **sourced from the kidney** nourishes the foetus. It determines the growing child's basic constitution, its strength and vitality. It forms the basis for growth development, sexual maturation and reproduction.

Conception and pregnancy are very much guided and controlled by jing and so where there is a kidney deficiency, and thus a jing deficiency then it is likely we will also see infertility and chronic miscarriage problems.

It moves in slow, mysterious cycles, presiding over the major developments in life. Again these cycles are explained in the Neijing and also in detail in the more well known, I Ching.

Female Jing Cycles of Seven

Age 7 - A girl's kidney energy initially begins to prosper at seven years of age (1x7).

Age 14 - Menstruation makes its first appearance as the *ren* (sea of yin) channel begins to flow and the *chong* (sea of blood) channel becomes stronger and begins to prosper. (2x7).

Age 21 - Her kidney *qi* balances and by now, she has a full mouth of completely developed teeth (3x7).

Age 28 - Thriving in her optimal condition, she exudes vital energy and her blood prospers. Her four limbs are strong and flourishing. (4x7).

From here, as we all know, it is *downhill*!

Age 35 - The *yang ming* channel depletes, her skin starts to dry and her hair begins to shed (5x7).

Age 42 - Her three yang channels, *tai yang, yang ming* and *shao yang,* all start to recede. Her complexion begins to deteriorate and there are the first appearances of grey hairs (6x7).

Age 49 The *ren* and *chong* channels are both receding, menstruation is ending. Her general physique is frailer and she can no longer conceive. (7x7).

(I am depressed to report I seem to be in the final cycle of my Chinese female life. It kinda feels like I might fall off the edge of the world soon...)

.

Anyone else depressed? Sorry girls! It's interesting how it corresponds though isn't it? Remember too, that rose supports kidney energy, and thus jing. This cycle then is entirely supported by the rose. Let's have a look now, at what that means for men. His cycle is different because it is measured not in 7 years, but in 8's.

Male Jing Cycles of Eight

Age 8 - A boy's kidney energy begins to prosper. His hair is well formed and lovely second set of teeth emerge at the age of eight (1x 8).

Age 1 6 - Kidney energy is growing now and he enjoys an abundance of vital energy. He is able to let his sperm out at the age of 16 (2x8).

Aged 24- Fully developed now, his kidney energy is strong and forceful. His extremities are well formed and powerful and all of his teeth are developed by now (3x8).

Aged 36 - Everything is strong and well formed and he is performing at his optimum power (4x8).

Now he will start to feel his decline.

Age 40 (*Of course, it is*!)
Energy starts to recede, as does his hairline and his teeth begin to fall out (5x8).
Age 48 - As yang energy of the entire body declines so his energy and drive does too. His complexion dries and withers and his hair begins to turn white. (6x8).
Age 56 - As kidney deficiency starts to kick in then liver energy cannot be sustained either. The connective tissues begin to suffer. The tendons become rigid and he is far less nimble than he once was. (7x8).
Age 64 - *When I get older, losing my hair….Will you still need me, will you still feed me….* The body is frail, hair is white and many teeth have been lost. (8x8).

So that's both sexes depressed now. I'm all for equality, y'all. Of course, the female jing cycle is far shorter because it pertains to how long she is fertile for.

Dried up and withered…pout.

Enough already!

Let's move on!

Spermatorrhea

Now that we have a comprehension of what jing is and how it affects us, it is easier to revisit the issues concerning spermatorrhea that I mentioned in the most fleeting manner in the write up about Cherokee rose.

I wanted to mention it in a section on its own because it is one of the fundamental areas where *western medicine and eastern medicine disagree*. In the west this trickle of semen is considered to be nothing more than a trifle with no real consequences at all besides a bit of tiredness and perhaps, a decline in sex drives.

In the 18th and 19 century Europe, however, doctors were not nearly quite as dismissive declaring it as a sign of all manner of character floors. By the 19th century spermatorrhea was widely regarded as having corrupting effects on the body. Treatment by a benign doctor was circumcision; on a bad day prescriptive treatment might even have been castration!

Today, though, it is mostly accepted as a *normal* part of a male's everyday life. Eastern medicines however, both TCM and Ayurveda take it incredibly seriously.

In Ayurveda it is considered to be a vata complaint and specifically they would treat it with winter cherry and country mallow.

In TCM, you might recall that the **worst strains on jing potency are semen, menstruation and pregnancy.** So then, this constant seeping of seminal fluid means that jing is consistently being wasted in the production of more. It is thought that spermatorrhea is caused by the **essence gate not being securely closed because spleen-kidney energy is not strong enough** or sometimes that **the essence chamber has been disturbed by an excess of dampness or heat.** Each time the essence gate opens, jing flows through, kidney power escapes which in turn reduces liver power too. Throughout this channel it means that most physical processes will be affected.

Treatment by TCM physicians is with Cherokee rose, or as it is sometimes also known Golden Cherry.

We see this idea of closing the essence gate many times throughout ancient writings about Cherokee rose, not only for seminal discharge, but also enuresis (excess urination) and excessive vaginal discharge too. Don't miss the connection too, that stress also reduces jing...so we would also see this as a way to treat stress related disorders.

Rose is a tonic for the kidney meridian. This is a yin meridian. That is: its energy flows upwards. Its role is to control growth and development of bones and to nourish marrow, which is the body's source of red and white blood cells. Here, you will see the blood alignment with jing.

Depleted kidney energy then, is often seen as a cause of both anaemia and of immuno-deficiency. Western medicine does not really have an equivalent for their “marrow” although it does include bone marrow, which obviously we do have, but marrow also encompasses the spinal cord and the brain too.

It follows then that poor memory, foggy headedness, an inability to think clearly, (and for those of you who have read my book on vetiver and The Professional Stress Solution, also of yin disease) are all regarded as indicators of impaired kidney function and deficient kidney energy. By the same token, since we are speaking of the spinal column, so does back ache too.

Looking at a person's complexion and hair usually gives a good external representation of kidney energy, (greasy, tired, toxic) as do the ears.

Tinnitus (ringing ears) is a sign of kidney dysfunction and also some of you who have read my other books, also of yin disease...

So along with the physical imbalances we expect to see with kidney meridian issues:

Chest pain, asthma, abdominal pain, irregular menstruation, impotence, hernia□

Blimey...apart from hernia and asthma, they all look frighteningly like a list to prescribe rose for, don't they? (And asthma might likely be up there if anxiety was known to be the trigger)

We are also going to see the emotional issues of

- Hysteria
- Paranoia
- Depression
- Fear

- Loneliness
- Insecurity

Emotionally, when in balance, good strong kidney energy presents itself as wise, rational, clearly perceptive, gentle and full of self-understanding.□

I think it is worth turning over a couple of our healing jigsaw pieces here. To do this I need to flash your minds back to some other books. **In the Essential Oils of the Mind Body Spirit** we talked about how fear was the emotion connected with the kidneys, and how "fear causes chaos in the qi. It is the energy of qi that both moves the essence and secures it. If fear causes a depletion of qi then the force of the essence depletes too". And yes, we will always see this fear/ kidney correlation happening whichever way we look at it. Whether it is an excess of dopamine being found in urine in veterans with PTSD to the little boy who has suffered trauma and is unable to stop wetting himself; it seems as though the two are most certainly inextricably linked.

Then the other jigsaw piece that seems to be important to me is how premature ejaculation is very much a yin disease, as seen in both the book on vetiver and also The Professional Stress Solution. Here, with the essence gate we find that we require yang energy to keep it shut. What reduces yang energy....stress and fear....

Round and around the healing carousel goes....where will it stop...? Only the goddess knows!

Chinese Medicine Usage of Rose

Typically treatment with rose in TCM is given as 3-6g of rosehips decocted into water for oral use. These might also be used by TCM doctors to calm heart and kidney complaints.

Rose petals are often used as additives into salads. To do this, wash well and allow to dry before tossing into your lettuce!

Rose hips are added to teas as are darker coloured rose petals.

Far more often than in the Western world, there is a strong usage of incense in China to promote emotional and spiritual balance. Respiratory complaints too, are treated with rose joss sticks.

By far the most popular of all the traditional medicine foods in China is ***congee,*** which is like a medicinal porridge or rice pudding. The very first a mention of this national treasure was by Emperor Huang I in his Zhou book. Today congee has become the prominent staple of the Tamil people.

Rose sugar too, is a quintessential part of Chinese life. The rose petals are spread onto a tray then dried until they are withered. Then they are slightly kneaded by hand and then mixed equal parts with sugar and kept in an airtight container until it can be used for cakes or teas.

Recipes for both rose sugar and congee can be found later in the book.

Chapter 5 Rose in Aromatherapy

In aromatherapy, we use two species of rose.

Rosa damascena – The Damask Rose, sometimes referred to as the Bulgarian or Turkish Rose

Rosa centifolia - The rose of a hundred petals, The Cabbage Rose or sometimes referred to as Rose de Mai. This is the same oil used in Ayurveda and that we also see in the ancient Greek and Unani writings of old.

Two main products are used: essential oil and absolute. Both of these can be found of both damascena and centifolia so check your labelling carefully.

- The essential oil is the product of distillation. You will see this labelled as Rose Otto or Attar of Roses. Otto is colourless and semi-solid in cooler conditions. Its fragrance is sweet and mellow and has a slightly clove-y and vanilla nuance to it.

- The absolute is not quite as heady as Otto. It is honey-golden and is more viscous than the attar. It seems to have a much spicier note. To me, the absolute has a warmer and more intoxicating feel to it.

Safety Data:

Rosa damascena

Tisserand and Young 2013 suggest a maximum topical dilution of 0.6%

Rosa centifolia

Tisserand and Young 2013 suggest a maximum topical dilution of 2.5%

Contraindications - Please avoid using rose essential oil as soon as you suspect you may be pregnant. Safe usage is only after 37 weeks.

Botany

The Rosa genus is enormous, encompassing 100 or more species and thousands of subspecies. The oldest known rose still in existence is *Rosa gallica* which probably dates back to about 12th Century BC. It is likely that gallica was potentially the rose of antiquity we recognise today.

The Damask rose that gives us Rosa damascena is most likely a descendant of this early gallica rose.

Rosa centifolia, you might sometimes see listed as Rose de Mai or Cabbage Rose. Its other name Hundred Petal Rose gives away its beautiful form, and they are indeed arranged in a way that makes the flower look like a delicate pink cabbage.

For the most part, early roses grew wild, and although we see them being cultivated in Rome and in China, this did not really become that widespread until the 17th century. Then, many new species were introduced to Europe, most notably the Chinese Tea Roses in the 19th century.

These new species improved the commercial viability of the rose greatly. The China roses would flower repeatedly, which was almost unheard of in the West. (The only species that did repeat flower seasonally was, interestingly enough, the Autumn Damask). They improved the fragrance too, bringing stronger and headier notes to the bloom. These Hybrid Teas, as they came to be known, also had a great range of colours extending the hues of roses for the garden from red and pink to whites, yellows and oranges.

The classification of a rose depends on having a woody stem. They can be erect, climbing or trailing. Their leaves grow alternatively on the stem, are usually serrated and can sometimes have prickles on the underside. Most of the species have five petals (although *Rosa sericea* has only four). Beneath the petals are four sepals and roses in nature are insect pollinated.

Extraction

Distillation

I've chosen to describe the extraction process as you would find it Saudi Arabia, mainly because there is more data to draw from about the artisan process, as opposed to the massive vats of Bulgaria and Turkey for instance.

That said the process is similar across the world. Historically, of course, rose attar was originally a bi product of the massive rosewater industry.

The rose comes into bloom in the Highlands of Al-Jabal and Al Akhdar between March and mid May. The region whose name means *Green Mountain* stretches between altitudes of 7,000 - 9,000 ft high

Pickers rise at dawn and pluck flowers until around 8am, where, at that point the blooms will be too open and begin to disperse their oils into the air. Picking early guarantees the largest yield of oil possible.

The rose blooms are collected onto a clean sheet of cloth and then are sealed into bags to ensure that none of the oils escape. Then when they arrive at the distiller they are strewn across a shed floor and are spritzed with rose water, to air them and ensure they do not begin to ferment.

The rose petals are the processed into ovens called Al-dhujans to dry the petals, and then placed in a vessel called Al-Burmah where they simmer gently for about 4 hours. Al Burmah is covered by a copper vessel (Qars) where the steam collects and then is cooled and condensed in a separate copper (Salha).

Fresh petals are then added to first waters and boiled. Then the rose water is left for 30 days to settle.

This process is how the rose oil would have originally been extracted for around 600 years, but it is thought that the double distillation process was introduced in Europe around the fifteen or sixteen century.

Double Distillation or Cohobation

During distillation, one vital ingredient is left behind - phenyl ethyl alcohol –which is slightly water soluble and is one of the main components that make up the lovely rosy fragrance of the essential oil. To draw this component back into the oil, the waters then go through a second distillation. This process is known as cohobation.

As well as using stream distillation, rose essential oil can also be extracted by using solvent extraction (Hexane), and high-pressure CO2 techniques.

Absolutes

Initially the petals are placed into a cylindrical drum along with an organic solvent, hexane. The drum is rotated to help the hexane to disperse and to separate the oil from the petals. This is then vacuum distilled to remove the solvent, which can then be recycled and used again. The waxy compound left behind is called a concrète or resinoid.

A "washing" utilises ethanol (pure alcohol) which then separates the aromatic compounds from the solid mass, and is then filtered. Finally the product goes through vacuum distillation one last time to retrieve the alcohol and to leave a pure essential oil.

Concrete

The same amount of petals will make 10 times as much concrete than essential oils. It is a very useful commodity because this solid mass can be placed in storage until the plant is ready to put it through the second stage to wash it.

Concrètes are used in other parts of the cosmetic industry but are rarely advertised for aromatherapy use because they are quite difficult to use - however you will sometime see benzoin concrète advertised. It comprises around 50-60% rose absolute.

Rose Wax

Many of the solids separated off in processing concrètes are waxes. This rose wax is also a saleable commodity and makes a beautiful emulsifier to creams and lotions. Safe usage is usually to roughly 10% of your final product. Whilst they make a lovely constituency to soaps, they are probably not much more than an expensive luxury here, because unlike in creams, the rose scent is not really strong enough to sustain itself.

Actions of Rose:

- Antidepressant
- Anti-inflammatory
- Antiseptic
- Antispasmodic
- Antiviral
- Astringent
- Bactericidal

- Choleretic (promotes the secretion of bile in the liver; to helps shed toxins from the body)
- Cicatrisant (forms scar tissue)
- Depurative (purifying and detoxifying)
- Emmenagoguic (stimulating blood flow to the pelvis. Esp. helpful to stimulating periods)
- Haemostatitic (curbs blood flow)
- Laxative
- Sedative
- Stomachic
- Tonic
- Uterine

So where should I start with my beloved rose?

I like to see results in my work. Strong measurable and obvious results so I think the way rose best does this is through its actions on the skin.

Skin care

Rose literally pours hydration into the complexion. It brings back a bloom that often seems long left behind. For me, it has always been rose absolute which is the oil of choice, because I adore the honeyed hue that it brings to a cream. Lately though, research has shown me that I might be wrong doing that, and that rose Otto should be the one to choose. The chemistry of the two, you will find later is quite markedly different. The absolute is rich in phenyl ethyl where the distilled oil has larger levels of citronellal and geraniol. It is citronellal that hydrates the skin so beautifully.

Because it is very cooling, rosewater makes the perfect skin toner. It is astringent and tightening to the skin and is deeply cleansing in the pores. Refreshing spritzes make lovely summer gifts and mums in labour with especially love you for these.

Rose is a very gentle oil, powerful, but gentle. We can trust it with sensitive skins and also very inflamed ones from rosacea and eczema.

For the most part we are looking at normal and dry skins here, sensitive and combinations and those complexions that are starting to lose their fertile glow.

Veins

Rose is superb for thread veins and also complexions that are starting to look compacted. You could use it for varicose veins but I find geranium to be a cheaper but more effective tonic here.

The action of rose here though, is to encourage the circulation to move. Remember the TCM ideal of fighting stasis? Cellulitis and generally bad circulation are both improved, especially with the addition of spices such as black pepper and ginger.

Heart medicine

Physically we think of palpitations and irregularities, but also emotional heart medicine too.

Congested Liver

I think this should come with a codicil. The liver is probably the most congested organ in the body. Stress, environmental toxins, drugs (prescription of other wise) and food all affect the liver. If there is a suspicion of depleted energy, because of outward symptoms of depleted kidney energy (as we see in the TCM section) then, yes, use rose. For cleansing the liver per se though, rosemary, eucalyptus and peppermint would all work better (*See the Essential Oil Liver Cleanse*)

Hormonal Imbalance

Whether this pertains to post natal hormones, menstrual cycles or menopause, rose is always our best friend. It eases both tension and bad moods but also as you will see later in the evidence it is wonderful for reducing pain. I would also use rose to pull irregular periods into a better cycle too.

There is strong clinical evidence that premenstrual problems and pelvic pain syndrome are made worse by the sufferer having previously experienced some kind or trauma or abuse. Most obviously we find women who are suffering from PTSD have a terribly painful menstrual pain. Rose is most definitely a liberating elixir for her.

Digestive

Constipation and nausea are both very well helped here.

Earache

I am a bit frightened of earache; it never bodes well and I think it should always be looked at by a doctor just in case. The pain though, can be managed with a rose and saltwater compress. Fill a pudding basin with hot water and dissolve a tablespoon of salt into it. Add one drop of rose. Soak a small compress in the water and squeeze it out. Place the warm pad over the ear. (*Over* the ear, mind; my old dad said you should never put anything smaller than your elbow *in* it...!)

Eyes

Sore eyes, itchy eyes, tired eyes...rosewater compresses or cold rosehip teabags!

Psychosomatic Illness

I opened the book with a quote from an enigmatic song by Suzanne Vega. It says:

"I'd like to meet you in a timeless, placeless, place...Somewhere out of context and beyond all consequences..."

We'll look at that more in depth in the spirituality section, but I feel this is very much the medicine of rose. It is a perfect treatment stress or trauma related incarnations of emotions experienced a long time before. Sometimes they can manifest so long afterwards there seems to be no context at all with the original pain. I think particularly of the female Gulf survivors who come back to normal life only to become the statistic of "twice as likely to suffer period pains". The same applies to those women who have survived domestic violence. The hurt no longer has context and it shows itself much later when the body now feels safer. There are no longer *consequences* for that "weakness"

If there seems to be no reason for pain, then meditation (or hypnotherapy) and rose are the very best prescription, used with cistus or amber to lift the trauma.

Be ready with handkerchiefs and the number of a good counsellor.

Sensuality

I don't know what it is about rose, but it just makes you feel good. More than that it makes you feel *ooh – la- la*! There is a happiness to it, a flirtiness almost, and the goddess connections are impossible to ignore. I suppose the tonic effects on the uterus are might have a part to play too. It is a bit like having an endless massaging of your sexual organs...and I'm all up for that!

Traditionally we say it is a woman's medicine, and it most certainly *is*, but later in the book you will find some rather remarkable data that I hope will make more people consider it for men.

We don't know *why* sexuality switches on and off, but I think psychologists would agree that there is a real for self esteem requirement for it to function well. How that actually translates into neurotransmitters has not really been fully answered yet.

What we do know is that trauma will slam the door on intimacy, and where we can see connections between the heart and intimacy, and then rose performs very well. In his book *Aromatherapy Healing the Spirit* Gabriel Mojay describes rose as "recommended for a loss of self-esteem of the very deepest kind-where emotional pain has injured the capacity for self-love....particularly for the resentment that results from emotional coldness, rejection and betrayal."

This is very powerful medicine indeed. Add any leakage of jing into the equation and sensuality might very easily be restored

Despair

Imagine roses laid onto a grave. Blood dripping from self harm wounds in the wrists. Safe hate because the love of your life has left you. Deep sadness at the realisation of the impossibility of a child. Wretched anxiety about bailiffs arriving at the door. The stricken horror of a bomb going off in front of you. The guilt at having laid that bomb...

If the pain is too raw to bear, then there is only one possible medicine and that is rose.

Even more dangerous than those which make us cry, is the anguish we silently hide away. We avert our eyes and try to forget the festering lesions buried there. These are the demons that go on to cause psychosis, eating disorders, alcoholism and even heart attacks if they are not eventually faced. Rose lets the wound run gently clear, releasing the congealed rot that has infected the spirit for so long.

It calms hostility and it lets you move on. Rose says...*it is what it is*. We feel like we are dying now...but I promise you spring will soon be here. And with this rebirth comes new strengths, new qualities and skills, for it is through challenge that we are changed.

And you know what they say...What doesn't kill you makes you stronger!

When you reach the clinical trials section you will discover that researchers now understand *how* rose makes the skin look younger. It works through the mechanism that controls cell growth. I deeply feel that energetic medicine of rose works on that emotional and on the same spiritual dimension too. Its energy enables us to build a new stronger sense of "I". Fresher, independent and stronger, but also far more compassionate too.

The normal outcomes of such heartache *should* be cynical, angry and bitter. And for most people they are. But with the sweetness of rose, that simply is not so. The heart relaxes, unfurls and warms, eagerly waiting for the next chapter of life to unfold.

Rose Hip Carrier

Clearly with a little imagination you could be using all manner of homemade carriers for your oils. In the How to Make section, you might create your own rose petal maceration for instance. Rose floral waxes make sublime additions to creams and lotions, but for actual carrier oils to buy...there is only really rose hip carrier.

I love it.

It is rich with a golden pinkie hue. It is so thick with vitamin C that you can almost taste it in your mouth as your pour it onto your hands.

Use it for nourishing the skin and also reducing hot angry inflammation. It is great for mature skin because it plumps and smoothes fine lines and wrinkles. Most important is its healing effects on scarring, and when mixed with helichrysm or jasmine it becomes an almost alchemical balm.

The cooling rose effect means it is a superb way to treat sunburn but also radiation burns from cancer treatment too. Conversely, I wouldn't use it on burns from the cooker etc though, because the oil will begin to fry on your skin!

I would also avoid it if I were treating a younger complexion, especially those more prone to acne. It is just too thick and you are tempting pore blockages I feel (Jojoba or camellia work better here.)

Rose oil blending note

Middle

Rosa damascena accounts for 90% of the absolutes and essential oils used in the perfumery industry, with centifolia making up the other 10%.

Rose blends well with:

Again this would be too long a list because damascena and centifolia blend well with most oils, but in my opinion particularly well with cedarwood, lemon, geranium and sandalwood.

It is useful to recall the wisdom from the third century BC that Theophastrus gave us earlier about rose: *"being very delicate and acceptable to the sense of smell, by reason of its lightness it penetrates as no other can and fills up the passages of the sense"*

Be sparing with your expensive elixir...it can overwhelm.

Chapter 6 The Rose Oil Industry

There are a couple of statistics that will be useful to help you to visualise the vast scale of rose oil industry.

Firstly: the size of the essential oils global statistics as a whole.

In 1990 the essential oils market was estimated to be worth US$616-million. By 2005 that figure had increased to $3.6-billion. According to the United Nations Comtrade statistics, the size of essential oil fragrance and flavour global market, by 2011, was estimated at US$ 24 billion and to be growing at an annual rate of 10 % year on year.

It is estimated that 0.01% (250,000 hectares) of the planet's agricultural land is given over to the production of essential oils.

Secondly:

One hectare of land can produce 3.5 to 5 tons of rose flowers, which will then be turned into 1kg of oil. That same quantity of flowers can also be used to make 10 times more concrète than oil.

The major producers of rose essential oil

To me, it seems to be only fair to begin by talking about Iran, who has provided by far the most scientific research included in this book. Until the 16th century Persia was the largest exporter of rose oil. Today, their export figures cannot match those of Bulgaria and Turkey but their influence through the rose continues to better our planet by providing inspiring and remarkable studies into the chemical and physiological effects of the oil.

However....

The main Rose producing countries are Turkey, Bulgaria, Iran, Morocco, India and China.

Bulgaria is viewed as the historical birthplace of rose oil, having produced essential oils for over 330 years. Their mantle as largest global producer was lost around the time of the Second World War, when the communist regime nationalised distilleries and insisted they were run under their supervision. (Some were returned to the rightful families after the fall of the regime in 1992)

Today, production in Bulgaria exceeds 6,000 tons of oil per year.

The production area is known as Rose Valley. It is situated in the centre of Bulgaria near Karlovo, Kalofer and Kazanlak and rose bushes grow in furrows as we in England grow potatoes! The combination of the soil and climate makes for perfect conditions for production of a stunning crop of roses with the optimum yield of oil.

Today, Bulgaria's Rose Valley boasts 3600 hectares of rose bushes (10,763 acres – thank you, Google) producing some 1.5 tons of rose oil every year.

Most of the oil produced in Bulgaria is headed for France to be used in perfumery. A slightly smaller volume is sold to the US. The next largest export market heads to Germany currently – for production of natural medicines. Japan also buys oil from Bulgaria for their food supplement marketplace. Many Bulgarian companies also produce rose oil exclusively for the Dubai perfumery market and are wholly financed by these fragrance firms who recognise the potential of the exquisite oil and are willing to pay large sums of money to enjoy a monopoly of it.

As much as 95% of the rose oil produced in Bulgaria is exported with the remainder being made into tiny vials of oils for tourists. (PS If you haven't discovered this yet, put the term "Muskal" into Ebay and it brings up these vials in beautiful traditional wooden packaging. Whilst I can't attest to quality because I have not seen a GC report, the fragrance is out of this world!)

Turkey

Today, Turkey holds the title of number one producer of Rose for the perfumery industry, with about 8,000 tons of flowers being harvested every year. Production stretches across fields through around 60 villages in the mountainside regions of Isparta, which is located just north of Antalya in the SW of the country. There, from the coast it has also grown into. Afyon, Denizli and Burdur.

It is estimated that Turkish rose production area equates to area is around 2300 (5683 acres) of which around half is found in Isparta. The plants are arranged into families and because of the variations in altitude that the roses grow at, it can mean that the harvest season is increased to almost double the time. Where in Saudi, the Taif season is just three weeks; here in Isparta it can run to seven or sometimes eight weeks. (The economic impact of this is phenomenal because it does not only mean that production is far larger, but of course there is more paid out in wages that will circulate back into the surrounding community).

Here there are two major species of rose cultivated for oil: Both Rosa damascena, the red damask rose and Rosa centifolia.

Getting the maximum yield of oil from your flower is a major determinant of whether your product will be financially viable or not. A minimum yield should be above 1 kg oil per 5,000 kg flowers, with a target in the range 3-3,500 kg flowers per 1 kg oil, but in these areas yield can vary hugely at anything from 1500- 10000 kg of flowers per1 kg of oil

Total production from Turkey is estimated at around 1.5 tonnes of rose oil and 7 tonnes of concrète (by comparison, Bulgaria is estimated to product around 1.5 to 1.8 tonnes of rose oil annually).

Export values currently at a peak of US$12.6 million (2012, most recent available data) but usually fluctuate between $8-12 million. Rose accounts for arountd50% of essential oil exports out of Turkey. As ever, France is their best customer buying up around 70% of all rose oil produced with European markets and US accounting for around most of the rest (22%).

Morocco

Comparatively Morocco is a far smaller producer, but is significant because it provides much of the industries maroc absolute.

Predominately we find most growers located in southern Morocco around El Kelaa M'Gouna, east of Ouarzazate. Here, different to the "potato field" imagery, the planting is far more romantic with rose bushes being used to mark the borders of cultivated plots of land along the banks of the M'Gouna and Dra Rivers. This is probably a throwback to the early need to work close to a natural water source for the oil production. The Moroccan Rose blossoms late in April but has a very low yield of oil, hence the development of the absolute.

Two emerging essential oil players are Saudi Arabia and Pakistan.

Saudi Arabia

Saudi Arabia has long enjoyed their Taif rose but it is only very recently that investment has been channelled into producers with a view to encouraging export.

Taif perfumers produce an annual export of around 75 kilograms (165 lbs) of pure oil each year—one twenty-fourth as much as Turkey produced in 1997.

The US / Arab oil relationship continues as it does in crude oil! The United States purchase about 40% of Saudi rose oil produced, Western Europe about 30 % Japan 7% with the other 23% being spread across "rest of the world" markets.

Pakistan

Emphasis in development in Pakistan is more focused on Rosa centifolia. In recent years their trade in commodities of wheat and food crops has suffered difficulties and so the government is appealing to farmers to turn to a more profitable stock.

The climate in Faisalabad produces fantastic flowering conditions for centifolia right through the year. The average single plant produces an astonishing 1000g of flowers during a year making this a very profitable crop.

Chapter 7 Rose Colour Meanings and Effects

The difference in rose colours has fascinated people for generations. In days gone by, elaborate messages were communicated through bouquets, as each species of plant translated its own vocabulary.

Flowers colours do make a difference to the scent of a rose, but also to its medicinal benefits. It feels like we should have a variety of oils from different roses so we can experiment and investigate other properties, but commercially this is unviable to do. A consumer wants a rose oil that smells like a rose...and over the years we have conditioned our minds to recognise a rose that is pink. Any other colour simply wouldn't sell!!!

One way to harness the colour energy of the rose is to make a rose *vibratory essence*. These are waters that have soaked up the healing energies of the plant. This way we can make a medicine that is exactly matched to the emotional challenges we face. I have attached directions about how to make a flower essence later in the book.

Here we look at the meaning and the vibration of the medicines growing in your garden.

Red rose

Meaning – Passionate love

Healing vibration:

Probably the easiest to remember, this is the colour of bloodshed, and in the same way it is the essence that helps us to face the wounds which we might have hoped had already healed. These are the injuries that, on the surface, seem to have gone but beneath are festering and screaming for attention. Its compassionate medicine reaches out as a salve for guilt that underlies the perception of pain. You might consider the parents who simply cannot switch off grieving for their child for fear of a sense of betrayal. The pain is real, but their perception of guilt makes it far worse for them to deal with.

The red rose is a thread through the infinite lifetimes of being. It is eternal and never ending and can connect in a timeless fashion, unhindered by space and time. (Remember timeless, placeless place...) Here we might think of the remaining fear from PTSD or grief, but it might also talk of a karmic lesson. The type of memory that belongs to another phase of the soul's development which remains unchallenged throughout this or other incarnations

This idea of "I can't look" for fear of disturbing some terrible pain is very much a coping mechanism designed to suppress feelings. Often we might see addiction, compulsion and obsession filling the void where facing that pain should be. Self hating strategies stack up layer on layer and form a fiercely angry welt that red rose energy is supremely good at dissipating.

Drama too; this creation of a "look at me" dynamic, is in keeping with the "Because I can't dare to" avoidance. Often this can translate into sexually deviant and dangerous behaviour. Narcissism, sexual compulsions, promiscuity are all signature traits here. Red roses can diplomatically draw the safety curtain down on the most aggressive performances, gently aligning sexuality with the soul pathway and removing it out of the angry arsenal of weapons that belong to the head. It draws out trauma, lays it gently open for the spirit to comprehend and then silently cleans and disinfects the emotional wound.

This is root chakra energy, sex and foundations. It is the healing gateway from those lessons learned in the first seven years of your life, of dependency, security and having your emotional needs met.

Yellow Rose

Meaning: Gladness, friendship, and promise of a new beginning, but it can however also convey jealousy.

Vibration: Emergency medicine of the solar plexus chakra! When someone suffers a trauma, eventually the shock to the tissues will start to change how the body acts at a cellular level, slowly driving up inflammations and markers of chronic disease. Yellow rose energy is first aid, slap bang; stop it in its tracks. It entirely dissipates the trauma before it has a chance to infect.

Pink roses are heart chakra energy:

Bright Pink Rose

Meaning: Appreciation and Gentleness

Vibration: This is truly the colour of the female consciousness as it stands today. It is the essential "widget" for anyone who dreams of manifesting an altruistic role but somehow always sees their goal slip away. Maybe connected, maybe not, is the quality of making time count! The pink rose (which, of course, is also damascene or centifolia essential oils) will seriously kick your ass if you are wasting time or managing it ineffectively. The medicine might be subtle, but with her 6ins Louboutains on her fragranced feet, you sure are going to feel it when she does. If you want to manifest, then goddess knows you most certainly *will*. Be warned though, if life can't get any fuller, then something will have to go. Make sure you say your goodbyes compassionately.

The pink rose is sisterhood, grace and your place in the cosmic order. How do you fit into the universe's plan and who can you call on to help you? Rose will tell you who, what, why where and when, and the chances are she will also present your purpose right there at your feet!

Prepare to leave those days of checking facebook every 20 minutes firmly behind you because the pink rose awakens purpose, she pulls together coincidences, and she plumps up the usefulness of every one of your talents until you are riding the crest of a tidal wave of dreams come true.

Pink rose energy draw out everything you were ever born to be.

Pale Pink Rose

Meaning: Grace, but also "Please believe me"

Vibration: Before any real healing can take place in the heart, or success starts to manifest through your life, there absolutely has to be some semblance of self esteem.

The pale pink rose is very good at helping you to like what you see in the mirror. It carries the gift of acceptance and unconditional self love. More than that though, it fosters healthy interpersonal connections.

Where the bright pink rose draws the dynamos to you, the movers and shakers who can help you carve your way; the soft pink rose governs your emotional support network, those people who can always be relied upon to view you with a compassionate embrace and to temper the effects of negative personalities around you.

Where red rose makes you peel back the sticking plaster that has been concealing festering wounds, the pale pink rose is gentler, releasing heart pain and trauma like a tiny boat set upon the millpond. Gently it simply drifts out of sight.

Green Rose

Rarely seen, there is a green rose, Chinensis viridiflora, but I can find no language meaning for it

Vibration:

This is heart chakra and the guardian of the pain gateway. The one that smacks shut when someone is hurt and trust, compassion and love are left out in the cold, freezing on the other side. Green rose is the careful little imp opening the door ajar and taking sneaky peek to see if the coast is clear. Over time, the door opens a little wider and stays open longer gradually allowing withered emotions to step inside of the heart for a warm.

Orange rose

Meaning: Desire, Enthusiasm

Vibration:

This is very clear bright sounding throat chakra medicine. It enhances creativity, it clears emotional blocks and it eases anger. It is quite a gushy energy this one. Imagine your mum at graduation flinging her arms around you in pride. That barrow load of energy is very much orange rose. It is happy, feisty, energetic and really, caught up in the moment, like nothing else matters.

Purple

Meaning: Enchantment

Vibration:

This is transient and transcendent energy of the third eye. A snapshot into another realm. It is intuitive, psychic and spiritual.

White Rose

Language: Purity, silence, innocence

Vibration:

This is the rose of the crown chakra, gently nurturing and compassionate. White rose essence engenders will to live and a commitment to see life's trials through to their resolution.

Chapter 8 - Evidence of Rose Medicine from Clinical Trials

I have changed the format of how this section looks. I hope you do not mind. I wasn't happy with the way the print screens looked, of the clinical trials. They were blurred and offended my OCD! Whilst I had referenced all trials in the bibliography, it still felt a bit hit and miss to me, if you wanted to refer to a trial in your own research or case histories.

So...

In *this* book, I have posted **a link to each study** so you can access it directly if you want to. Please feel free to say you love it or hate it in the reviews of the book so I can get some idea of whether it should stay or it should go.

As ever, I'll start with a reminder that **an extract of rose oil might not necessarily mean an essential oil, or even the absolute, has been used for a clinical trial**. Over the next few pages we see petals, rose hips, aqueous and ethanoic extracts all being used. This is purely because the particular method used is deemed to be the best for isolating a certain constituent or biological action to prove its worth. Likewise, it also important to remember that, for some of the cancer studies in particular, these are very early, preliminary studies in test tubes and on rodents...**we still do not have proven cures for human cancer yet**. Also, remember that **not every chemical constituent of the rose passes through distillation or solvent extraction**, so whilst this helps us understand what the rose can do, it does not entirely validate what the *essential oil* or the *absolute* can do. To me though, it does seem like we can agree that the rose medicines from strain to strain (damascene, centifolia, Cherokee etc) each has the same scope of properties to a greater or lesser extent

The race is very clearly on to find these elusive diabetes, heart disease and cancer cures, and regardless of the hype that some essential oils suppliers are giving, there is no "them and us" situation with the clinical researchers. When the active constituent is proven to cure cancer, the drugs companies will synthesize and patent it and we can all celebrate *together*. Please do not take any of these notes as the final declaration of cure...because as yet...we know of no such thing.

Having depressed the hell out of you now let me remind you that by the end of the book, you will know everything about rose that clinical researchers do in May 2015. Use your information wisely, get your bottle of oil out and set it to work. Remember the men in white coats are guided by TCM, Ayurvedic and Unani wisdoms; it is up to us to build and expand that knowledge so that our children's children can cite *us* as the healers that gave them their inspiration for the next stage of experiments.

Design new products, make candles and evaporators to lift the spirits of the unwell (remember from ***The Essential Oils of The Mind Body Spirit*** that we now know that the mood balance molecule serotonin influences how cancer cells travel through the body, for instance.) Get out there and make your medicine sing because ***we*** have always known that emotions affect the physical body and that positive thinking, forgiveness and a release of hostility are the best weapons we have against illness. Using aromatherapy that way...you are light years ahead of the laboratories and performing an extremely important job while the labs catch *us* up!

So...what have the men in white coats found so far...?

Menstrual Pain

I think is probably fair to say that one of the primary uses in aromatherapy, for rose is as a uterine tonic. It is blissful relief from period pains, a real ally in labour and a new mother's very best friend as it contracts the womb back to normal size. As therapists we also celebrate how it anchors that feeling of femininity that giving birth can steal.

The effects on the womb are well documented now and although most of these trials attest to the effects of dysmenorrhoea (painful periods) I have found rose to be effective, really, across all aspects of menstruation. It might be useful to just have a look at some of the other ways rose can be used here:

- **Metrorrhagia** - this is where periods have become irregular and no longer show a predictable cycle
- **Menometrorrhagia** - These unlucky ladies suffer from too many and very heavy periods
- **Polymenorrhoea** - this is when bleeding drops to intervals of less than 21 days making fertility almost impossible because the corpus luteal phase ,where

the body makes progesterone to protect a pregnancy, becomes almost non existent

- **Chronic Pelvic Pain Syndrome** - A complex disorder affecting both men and women in all aspects of the pelvic region from pain during sexual relations to problems with urination and excretion and even during exercise.

On average menstrual blood loss should be about 35-40 ml (1½ fl oz). Only about 10% of women report losing any more than about 80ml (2oz) during a cycle. Holistic medicine has a great deal to offer here because both menorrhagia and dysmenorrhoea are quite subjective terms, and really, orthodox medicine is not very well equipped in dealing with things that are not exact science! The term is not really a measurable one, **it pertains to the *emotional burden* of the flow**, or its pain being more than the patient feels she can comfortably deal with. **The National Institute for Health and Care Excellence (NICE)** defines heavy menstrual loss as ***"excessive blood loss that interferes with a woman's physical, social, emotional and/or quality of life"***

I'll begin by citing a work that does not come from a laboratory, but instead from a nursing study, done on actual ladies, by one of the most formidable aromatherapists of our generation.

Jane Buckle, author of *Clinical Aromatherapy; Essential Oils in Practice* is both an aromatherapist and a nurse (and a wonderful writer!). Potentially she has done more for the fight of getting clinical aromatherapy into mainstream hospital environments that anybody else. For the many numbers of you who ask about credible and trustworthy sources, Jane is most certainly one. Anyone who has a serious interest in understanding aromatherapy should read at least one of her books. Here, in a trial done with The School of Nursing in Ishkan, Korea she demonstrates how rose applied topically to the abdomens of a series of college students showed significant reductions in the pain of menstrual **cramps when used with clary sage and lavender** in comparison to the test subjects who received a placebo dose. I am surprised to see she opted for ***Rosa centifolia*** here, since I think most therapists might more likely gravitate to *damascena*. It is interesting to see the results seem to have been just as impressive.

This menstrual pain trial into Rosa centifolia can be found at: http://www.ncbi.nlm.nih.gov/pubmed/16884344

So, then, a trial done by the Iran University of Medical Sciences in Sept 2014 threw light on something that often occurs in aromatherapy. That is: a person will have an oil recommended to them, use it for a few days and then quickly lose interest/ faith in the remedy. Here, three groups of women were given treatments to use on the first day of their period over two successive cycles. The first group were given an almond massage oil with *Rosa damascena* added. The second group were given a blank almond oil, the third was given the instruction to self massage but not to use oil at all.

I was pleasantly surprised to find that the pain was reduced in *all* groups during the first cycle. (I was expecting to find no effects from simple massage without oil! How about that for a testimony into the power of touch?!!) The first cycle effect was low though, and listed as ***not significant***. However when the red flag started to fly for the second cycle the rose group all reported significant improvements in their pain experience.

I think this is a particularly important trial for two reasons. The first is that we see the proof that essential oil medicine is gentle, subtle but most of all cumulate. We know then that we might have to use rose for a number of weeks before we experience significant effects. (And we will see evidence of this again in later trials too). But also this "self massage" idea seems, to me, to be important. A woman can take care of her own femininity. That's empowerment in the very *truest* sense of the word but, also, it is potentially a massive relief to the health service burden. Costing around £7 million a year it is the second biggest reason for NHS gynaecological referrals in the UK.

http://www.ncbi.nlm.nih.gov/pubmed/25254570

Again, we have researchers from Iran to thank for this next study. This time it is the students from Kowsar dormitory in Tabriz University of Medical Sciences. All were aged between18-24, were single, had a BMI of between 19-24 and rated their menstrual pain on a scale of being between 5-8.

Each student was given an envelope which had been randomly chosen to either be rose or the more usual medication given for menstrual pain, *mefenamic acid.* The capsules had been made to look entirely identical and they were instructed to take them on two consecutive cycles, at 6 hour intervals for three days.

The results of the trial were almost identical in both groups, a slight improvement in pain in the first cycle and a significantly reduced pain experience in the second cycle, particularly in the first three hours. The treatments were both able to reduce the pain significantly right up to the third day when pain had virtually disappeared.

Rose then, offers an equally effective pain treatment, without the concerns of side effects that the synthetic mefenamic acid can carry...which incidentally are disconcertingly plentiful!

You can find this study into ***Rosa damascena*** at:

http://www.ncbi.nlm.nih.gov/pmc/articles/PMC3964428/

Pain Reducing (Post surgical)

But this pain mechanism is not confined to *uterine* pain. Rose seems helps the perception of physical discomfort right across the spectrum. (So perhaps we might find that this is not evidence of a uterine tonic, merely into a reduction in pain. It is hard to know yet.)

The next study is a beautifully detailed cross discipline trial by nurses in Isfahan University of Medical Science in Iran. It investigates how rose was used on very small children (aged between 3-6) after they had undergone surgeries, to assess how much difference the calming affects of rose would make to their *perception* of pain. Here, they were given rose essential oil to inhale and were compared to the placebo group who had been given almond oil to sniff. (Almond had been chosen because of its inclusion into other comparable trials and also because it has no respiratory effects that might distort the findings). The results were very favourable.

One to two drops of the oil were placed onto eye pads placed 30cm away from the patients head (presumably on their pillow) at periods of 3, 6, 9 and 12 hours post operatively. (They still had the usual post operative checks such as sedation, tablets to prevent infection high fever etc). The pain was then assessed 30 minutes after each aromatherapy oil dose, during a 5 minute observation by a researcher.

The first assessment, immediately upon arrival showed no difference between the groups, but post operatively the rose team always reported less pain, and the difference between the two groups grows more dramatic with each reading.

At 3 hours, the placebo group reported a mean pain reading of 2.6, but the rose patients were faring far better at just 1.03.

By 12 hours the placebo group are left standing with a mean pain score of 1.1, and rose having dropped to a pain score of just 0.4.

Incidentally, it is worth stating here, that there was a good cross section of different modalities of surgeries involved in this trial, from thoracic to gastric, which makes it harder to suggest that the effects of oil were happening because of a tonic effect of the digestive system etc.

You can find this trial at:

http://www.ncbi.nlm.nih.gov/pmc/articles/PMC4387651/

Sexual Dysfunction

To me this is the most glorious of the trials because it spotlights just how closely aligned orthodox and complementary medicine have become. Plus more importantly, I think, it spotlights male sexuality as opposed to the most usual female alignment we see with rose, and it also examines how the plant will affect a *physical* complaint with its roots in e*motional* dis-ease.

Even more exciting is that the research is, quite literally, global reaching from substance abuse researchers in Iran, to psychiatric units in Switzerland and addiction studies in Thailand.

You can find this trial at:

http://www.ncbi.nlm.nih.gov/pmc/articles/PMC4358691/

It investigates the effects of using rose extract on 60 male patients with a mean age of 32. Each was suffering from a Major Depressive Disorder (MDD) and was being prescribed SSRI's. Selective Serotonin Re-uptake Inhibitors are the most common type of antidepressant prescribed today. The problem is these SSRIs can have disturbing and distressing side effects on any or all phases of the sexual cycle. This might be through decreased libido, on impaired arousal, or causing erectile dysfunction; SSRIs are most commonly associated with delayed ejaculation and problems of delayed, or even absent orgasm.

Participants completed questionnaires about their mood and their sexual dysfunction at baseline recruitment commencing the trial, at 4 weeks and at 8 weeks. They were given a 17mg oral dosage of citronellol from the essential oil (2ml daily).

At four week, the effects were already beginning to become obvious. Both placebo and rose group were experiencing a lift in their mood and a slight improvement in sexual symptoms. By 8 weeks there was a significant difference between the groups. Whilst both groups were showing improvements with both erection and ejaculation by week 4; by week 8, both mood and sexual function was markedly improved in the rose group.

	A	B	C	D	E	F
Sexual drive	1.8	1.84	2.07	1.88	2.43	2.03
Erections	1.78	1.94	1.77	1.82	2.49	2.05
Ejaculations	1.89	1.92	2.01	1.88	2.71	2.20

Fig 1. Key:

Column A – Rose Baseline Reading

Column B - Placebo Baseline

Column C - 4 wk rose

Column D - 4wk placebo

Column E - 8 wk rose

Column F - 8 wk Placebo

So, now I am hoping the TCM researchers pick up this study and find how many of these many men with MDD are also suffering from spermatorrhea...Might this be the beginnings of proof of drainage of jing, I wonder?

Incidentally, I would presume that the oil in this treatment was administered in an essential oil capsule. I would not mimic it just yet, if only because of the cost (although clearly there are many other safety considerations) at an average of $40 for 2 ml you are looking to rack up a weekly bill of nearly $300 and nearly two and a half grand for eight weeks.

Let's face it...the sex would need to be pretty mind blowing for that level of investment really, wouldn't it?!

I'd get massaging instead if I were you. I'll leave location and technique to choice!

Skin

So, here now, I have one of those "where shall I put it in the book" dilemmas because the next report is about stress, *and* it's about the skin. In fact it is about how a team of researchers assessed the affects that stress had on a rat's skin, mapped the physiological process and then looked to see if rose could help. The short answer is "Hell, yes!!!" The long answer which I would prefer to impress you with is this...

Stress increases the release of Adreno corcotrophoid Hormone (ACHT) and also glucocorticosteroids. This is turn fires **H**ypothalamus, **P**ituitary, **A**drenal (HPA) axis and causes inflammatory effects in many areas of the body, but for the purposes of this trial, the skin because of mega doses of adrenaline, noradrenalin and cortisol being released into the system for too long a time.

The rose was proven to act directly with the brain increasing activity in a region called the *hypothalamic paraventricular nucleus* [PVN]) thus reducing this firing of the HPA axis, and then also to inhibit the manufacture of the plasma corticoids (which have been proven to be the nasties that cause stress related skin disturbance). It was also seen to prevent water loss from the skin (as well as increasing the saliva levels in their mouths, which *really is* hydration, isn't it!)

But the most incredible thing about this trial is the rose is not used topically...

Nuh-uh, not even!

All this was achieved simply by their inhalation of rose! Inhibiting the stress response had a direct affect on stress related skin disorder.

https://www.aromaticscience.com/effect-of-rose-essential-oil-inhalation-on-stress-induced-skin-barrier-disruption-in-rats-and-humans-2/

Sebborheic Dermatitis

Ok, so now to a very concise little report which explains how "0.01% extract of petals of ***Rosa centifolia***" (not sure if that is essential oil or not, even in the larger report it is unclear) is being developed by dermatologists in Korea, to make a shampoo for people with sebborheic dermatitis on the scalp. In particular they are looking for a weapon against the *malessezia* fungus that causes so many facial complaints.

For those of you who are not familiar with these conditions, one form of sebborheic dermatitis that most of us are familiar with is cradle cap (or cradle crap as my daughter Aimée referred to Dexter's bright yellow scale as!)

As the patient gets older the condition tends to start to present on the scalp as dandruff, then redness and irritation turning to increased scaling.

It usually begins on the scalp then wanders down the neck until it develops in the eyebrows, down the folds at the side of the nose, the face and the temples. The red flaking can be particularly troublesome behind the ears, where the greasy flakes get stuck in the patient's hair. If it finds its way into the ears and ear canal, it is called *ear eczema,* funnily enough. You might also find it in the folds under the breasts, armpits, and groin and between the buttocks. These are *sweaty* areas, basically, because the eczema is caused by a reaction of the sebaceous glands.

Scientists have now identified that this particular type or dermatitis always has a common link where this yeast spore *malessezia* is present on the skin.

The results from this trial were a bit of a mixed bag really, but with an aromatherapist's eye it is easy to suggest why this might be. The shampoo seemed to have a lovely effect on the lesions themselves but was disappointing in reducing the sebum production they had expected. (Rose nourishes not dries...) Mr Researcher Sir, I'd try some vetiver or ylang ylang in there for that if I were you!

Sebborheic trial into Rosa centifolia:

http://www.ncbi.nlm.nih.gov/pmc/articles/PMC4252671/

Acne

An interesting cross departmental discipline was conducted by **Yuangang Zu** et al. in 2010 where they assessed several essential oils against different bacteria. There is more mention of this trial in the bacteria section but here, it is useful to talk about the effects of **rose** against ***Propionibacterium acnes,*** bacteria thought to be responsible for the formation of skin acne. Thyme, cinnamon and rose essential oils showed the best inhibitory properties against this troublesome toxin. Very slight variations between the efficacies; rose came up top, but only just. Believe it or not, when the kill time was assessed in the test tube, each of the oils had battered the bacteria into submission is just *5 minutes* at a 0.25% dilution.

https://www.aromaticscience.com/activities-of-ten-essential-oils-towards-propionibacterium-acnes-and-pc-3-a-549-and-mcf-7-cancer-cells-2/

Skin Dryness

So that's acne, but for the most part I think most would agree that rose is more a treatment for skin *dryness* whether that be treating or preventing it. Researchers from the German University Medical Centre of Freiberg discussed this in a 2011 study where they tried to ascertain not only which extracts were useful, but also *why* they were.

They were able to ascertain that rose absolute seemed to contribute to keratinocyte differentiation, in other words how the protein cells in the base layer of the epidermis multiply and then gravitate to the surface of the skin, providing new fresh skin growth and helping to maintain a stronger (less flaky) skin structure.

http://www.ncbi.nlm.nih.gov/pubmed/20711260

Digestive

Constipation

I'll be brief.

Guinea pigs were given aqueous extract of *damascena* by researchers in Iran, and it caused their ileum to contract, leading the researcher to suggest it might be worth exploring as a laxative agent. Here though the effects were quite mild so this is a delicate ladylike lax, rather than the dynorod approach that I would rather be searching for.

http://www.ncbi.nlm.nih.gov/pubmed/25050281

But....

Hmmm...

Rattie rascals have thrown a spanner in the works because about nine months later, another team in Iran rosed up some rats in their trial to investigate the extract for gastro-intestinal problems. Here they discovered that the amount the intestine contraction was affected by a **relationship with the amount of extract the rats had**

been given. Further again, it seemed to be a *cumulative* effect. The amounts given were 500mg, then a 1000mg then 1500mg. Each dose added seemed to reduce the contraction (and thus the tummy ache) more.

Cleverly by 2013, this strange anomaly seemed to have explained by Sadraei et al. They were able establish **that it was the dosage** that had made the difference. There is no protecting you from the rat's demise here, since it is important to understanding the figure. The rats had been killed and then a section of their ileum had been put into Tyrone's solution to nourish it, then they stimulated it using electrodes.

Very low dose treatments of damascena, in *microgram* measures, had caused the ileum to contract. But when the dosage increased to *milligrams* then the smooth muscle relaxed and the contraction was inhibited.

Clearly, stating the dosage here is probably surplus to requirement since el-rattos ileum might be a tad smaller than your average human with gastric flu, plus the experiment was done with rose extract rather than essential oil, but in this case I think it safe to say, another drop or two in your tummy ache mix wouldn't hurt at all.

So, the scientists then set off to try and work out which active constituents were doing all the work here, and came to the conclusion that geraniol and citronellol were the big guns we have to thank.

Renal Colic

Yes, yes, I know renal colic is not the same as normal colic...but...

It's tummy cramps so....

Now this is nice because it adds weight to the TCM idea that rose affects the kidney meridian. It was done in what must be an incredibly busy emergency room which managed to recruit a massive 80 participants with renal colic. Both were given the standard orthodox treatment: (diclofenac sodium, 75 mg intramuscularly) half were given rose oil and half a placebo. Their pain was then assessed 10 minutes and subsequently thirty minutes later. As we can probably guess by now, ten minutes later there was little to choose between the two group's pain measures, but after thirty minutes....

All together now...

The rose group was better!

Their pain was significantly reduced in comparison to the placebo group.

Now I have to confess to not being as thorough as I should be with this one because the free access to the report just says rose *essential oil* but gives no indication of species, dose or method of administration. I am too tight to pay $51 to get access to this particular report to check this one point. If you feel the need, feel free to check at

http://online.liebertpub.com/doi/abs/10.1089/acm.2011.0941

Anti Bacterial

This next experiment sought to investigate the various antioxidant and anti bactericidal effects of damascene. But I also found it interesting because it includes both essential oil and absolute and then compares the relative constituents of each oil.

The absolute was found to contain 78.38% phenyl ethyl,

In the essential oil and hydrosol, citronellal and geraniol were found to make up a far larger percentage of the oil at more than 55%.

The total levels of phenols were found to be higher in the absolute and the essential oil than the levels found in the hydrosol.

The absolute and essential oil both showed impressive results in fighting strains of:

- **Escherichia coli** (ATCC 25922) - more commonly referred to as E- Coli, this bacteria lives in the intestine and is usually indicated in cases of food poisoning.
- **Pseudomonas aeruginosa** (ATCC 27853) –A nasty pathogen that multiplies in a number of environments, but most often in hospitals, and tends to attack people with weakened immune systems.

- **Bacillus subtilis** (ATCC 6633) A naturally occurring bacteria found in soil, but also in the human gastro-digestive tract, that causes vomiting and diarrhoea.

- **Staphylococcus aureus** (ATCC 6538), - Again, it exists naturally in the human respiratory tract, however is also responsible for skin break outs such as boils, for respiratory infections such as *sinusitis* and *impetigo,* and far more dangerous conditions such as *meningitis, pneumonia, endocarditis* and *toxic shock syndrome.*

- **Chromobacterium violaceum** (ATCC 12472) Causes potentially fatal *skin lesions and skin abscesses*

- **Erwinia carotovora** (ATCC 39048) - A crop pathogen that destroys root crops.

http://www.ncbi.nlm.nih.gov/pubmed/19688375

A 2010 report published in ***Phytotherapy Research*** put a bit of flesh on the bones of why rose was so effective against all of these horrible bugs. The researchers from the University of Szeged were interested in a phenomenon known *as* ***Quorum Sensing*** which is the way that pathogens swarm together to fight strongly enough resist antibiotics. Learning how to inhibit this sensing and swarming mechanism is a large part of being able to overcome the current problem of drug resistant strains to bacteria and this particular strain of research is coming up with dynamic strategies to overcome persistent and non treatable infections. The effects of essential oils were assessed against several bacteria strains including the precursor to E-Coli.

Most effective of the essential oils were found to be ***rose, geranium, lavender*** and ***rosemary***. Eucalyptus oils and citrus oils displayed moderate effects, but through a different physiological process. In the fight against quorum sensing camomile, juniper and orange were deemed to be ineffective.

https://www.aromaticscience.com/inhibition-of-quorum-sensing-signals-by-essential-oils-2/

Anti-diabetic

In 2009, a group of unlucky rats had diabetes induced, and were loaded up with maltose to skew their blood glucose levels. One set of rats were treated with *Rosa damascena* and the others were administered with ***acarbose*** a drug used to treat Diabetes mellitus II, and in some countries is also used to treat *pre*-diabetes. Oral administration significantly reduced the blood glucose levels found in the rats. The researchers from Kerman School of Medical Science in Iran stated that further investigation is warranted because the Rose extract had seemed to suppress the absorption of carbohydrates from the intestine and also to reduce to glucose levels after eating.

Diabetes evidence of ***Rosa damascena:***

http://www.ncbi.nlm.nih.gov/pubmed/19380218

Fat Reduction

Ok, so who has got their biology hat on? Because this one's a doozy!

If you are a cake monster like me though, you are ***going to want to know this.***

Cutting a very long-words story short, scientists from Tochigi in Japan found that extracts from ***R.centifolia*** were able to isolate certain enzymes in the blood that synthesize into the lipids that make us fat! Rose seems to target this *Diacylglycerol acyltransferase* by preference and then inhibit it, reducing the amount of adipose fat we produce. Adipose tissue's *specific job* is store fat in order to turn it into energy later. Interestingly they were also able to show that rose did not affect either liver or pancreatic activity, so now we know that this fat storage process actually takes place in the blood. This has led the scientists to suspect that it will be a useful way to treat metabolic disorders.

You can find this trial into ***Rosa centifolia*** at:

http://www.ncbi.nlm.nih.gov/pubmed/21538210

*But, a*s ever, just as we think we have found a plant healing happy place, the land of plant medicine shows itself to be is a strange and very confusing one. On one hand we find we might have found the eternal elixir for thin hips and all things cakeness then some mean scientist from the Physiology Research Centre in Kerman, Iran just has to go and spoil the fun. To give him his due, he might be saving the lovers of Red Velvet a heart attack or two, but it still seems a bit mean to me.

This time they used rabbits to demonstrate their point, and tested *Rosa damascena* and a plant called *Quercus infectoria*. This was a new plant to me, but it is an oak tree from Asia which apparently provides extraordinary medicine not that dissimilar to *damascena* in that it is digestive, and used for gyne problems (as well as toothache!). Their findings showed that giving Rosa damascena to a group of hyperlipidemic rabbits reduced the efficiency of left ventricular of the heart and its diastolic pressure, leading them to surmise that **using *Rosa damascena* with a high fat diet *may* lead to hypertension.**

So the waist size might decrease, folks, but it looks like we might be also investing in meters to check our blood pressure doesn't skyrocket too. Clearly, this is two different species of rose, but the rest of the properties of different species of rose seem so similar that I think we would be daft to discount this. It's not a scary blood pressure issue I don't think, but it does mean that we still haven't found a way to eat cake every day either!!!

How completely and utterly rubbish!

Should you want to download the report into ***Rosa damascena*** so you can stick pins in it... http://www.ncbi.nlm.nih.gov/pubmed/24163695

Epilepsy

I feel almost nostalgic writing up the next trial, because I mentioned it my free book *The Complete Guide to Clinical Aromatherapy and the Essential Oils of the Physical Body*. I found it, added it to the text and promptly lost it for three weeks where I nearly gave myself a coronary worrying about it....only to find I had already added the reference to the bibliography and forgotten it!!!

Hopefully it and I will fare better this time.

Basically we have furry friends fitting because they have been injected with ....something not very pleasant. They were then tested using a variety of different rose extractions, ethanoic extracts, aqueous extracts and chloroformic extracts.

Latency to the first minimal clonic seizure and generalised clonic tonic seizures were then recorded. To the rest of us, this means they measured how long the gaps were between the first and the rest of the seizures. Regardless of the extract the results were consistent, that the latent gaps between the seizures increases. The rats were fitting less often.

We know then that *Rosa damascena* has an anti-convulsive effect. As to how that works, well that remains a mystery thus far.

In 2008 this research was added to by Ferdowsi University of Mashhad, Iran who wanted to see whether rose could affect the onset of *early* seizures. Again we have rodent groups, this time they are having epileptic fits induced by electrodes on their brain. Those that had been given *Rosa damascena* had a significantly longer period until the onset of the first seizure in comparison to the control group. This leads to the suggestion that rose slows down the rate that the small electrical signals running through the brain gather momentum and cause a seizure. This is known as ***kindling acquisition,*** (so think of how small twigs can lead to a dangerous conflagration) it is thought that this is probably due to rose's impact on the GABA receptors - (which we'll come back to in a moment)

http://www.ncbi.nlm.nih.gov/pubmed/18819571

Heart medicine

I have got some very cool new words for you to use in your case histories

- **Inotropic** - The force or energy used in a muscle contraction
- **Chronotropic** - This is the speed of heart rate.

Both of these pertain to cardiac medicine. Unsurprisingly, given rose's strong associations with the heart, doctors in Iran wanted to understand *how*, exactly, it affects it? Here they were able to establish that rose probably stimulates beta-adrenoreceptors. These receptors are housed in the cell membrane of the heart and are affected by adrenaline. (You need to read the

HPA axis explanation in the sebborheic dermatitis trial to understand how this fires) and thus calm the stress related cardiac response.

Check the report at:
http://www.ncbi.nlm.nih.gov/pubmed/23688388

Also rose was found to affect the pathways of an enzyme **called 3-hydroxy-3-methylglutaryl-coenzyme**. *Its* job it to metabolise liver enzymes in the ketogenic and mevolanate pathways. Now the reason I found this particular piece of research interesting is that the mevolante pathway recognises and registers levels of cholesterol.

The metabolic process that occurs when **the body does not have enough glucose for energy** is known as **ketosis** and is registered in this ketogenic pathway. When this happens stored fats are broken down, which results in a build-up of acids called ketones within the body. Some people encourage this **ketosis** by following a diet called the **ketogenic** or low-carb diet. Interestingly, one of the foremost anti-epileptic treatments in use today is the ketogenic diet...and now we also find that an essential oil found to be effective for both epilepsy and cardiac complains can positively affect this pathway....

Here is the data to this particular jigsaw piece! http://www.ncbi.nlm.nih.gov/pubmed/20038104

Liver

Very quickly, scientists in India were able to show that *Rosa damascena* protects the livers of rats, mainly through its anti-oxidant properties.

http://www.ncbi.nlm.nih.gov/pubmed/23339694

Early promising cancer evidence

Right then hold onto your hats people, because this is about to get breathtaking...quite literally.

The following trial was undertaken in Chennai in Sept 2014 and it investigated the joint efforts of R*osa damascena* with nano particles of silver in the fight against lung cancer.

You can find the trial at:
http://www.ncbi.nlm.nih.gov/pubmed/25312140

Lung cancer cells, adenocarcinoma A459, were subjected to a mixture of silver and rose in what is known as a MTT Assay. This is a colour test where the addition of a new mixture should demonstrate the activity happening in the test tube by a change of colour. In this case the cells changed from light yellow to brownish yellow. The activity showed that the solution of silver and rose started to surround the cancer *cells in less than one minute,* and then to overcome the cells in an extraordinarily short time frame.

So now it's the turn of Egypt to put their rose deck on their table, and it is wonderful to see that they have specifically focused on the Taif rose for their investigations, but even more interestingly they have compared the effectiveness of different extractions on cancer cells, in particular the concrète and the absolute.

Both the concrète and absolute oils demonstrated cytotoxic activity against two kinds of human cancer cell lines: **HepG2** which you will probably guess is a **hepatic cancer** cells which cause changes to the liver and **MCF7** which is a **breast cancer cell**. When comparing how effectively the rose did its job, the concrète showed an inhibitory concentration (IC50) of **16.28** and **18.09** µg/ml, respectively**. The absolute was more efficient in reducing the activity** though. The inhibitory concentration of HepG2 was 24.94 and for MCF7 19.69.

This paper can be found at: http://www.ncbi.nlm.nih.gov/pubmed/24101441

Then in 2013 a superb paper was published, again in Iran, into the effects that *Rosa damascena* had on a specific colon cancer cell SW742. Colon cancer is the single biggest cancer threat in the US today. To compound the problem, orthodox treatments such as chemotherapy, surgery and radiation treatments all carry their own set of side effects. The race to find plant treatments here then is fiercely competitive.

So *Rosa damascena* was tested on cancerous cells but also fibroblasts in test tubes,

Now, how much did you take in when you read the essential oil extraction part? Can you remember that rose oil goes through a process called cohobation, because the water soluble part of the oil including *phenol ethyl alcohol* is left behind in the first distillation, so then it has to be processed again to put it back?

Ok, so the study found that the water soluble part of the rose oil caused the cells to multiply (cell proliferation).

But by contrast, the *non soluble* parts of the oil *inhibited* cell proliferation.

I think you might enjoy this report: http://www.ncbi.nlm.nih.gov/pmc/articles/PMC4017490/

Chapter 9 The Effects of Rose on The Mind

I am quite sad to say that, as yet, there seems to be no proof into the areas I think are the most useful areas for rose. I passionately hope this is not because they are not being researched. To me, and every other rose oil user before me is no oil to touch rose against the heartache of grief. No-one understands yet, what neurochemistry happens when we grieve. I can't imagine that knowledge is now far away. I can't help but wonder how similar the affects will be to *drug* withdrawal for instance. Or will we see that grief triggers the beta adrenoreceptors of the heart...which we already know that rose does too. What we do know for certain, but have no evidence to support it - except for hundreds of years use - is that rose helps reduce the heartbreak of grief.

In the same way, I have seen the affects of rose on PTSD to be astounding. It gently opens the wound allowing the pain to crawl out and then simply watches as the sharpness of the memory dissipates. We do have considerable evidence now of the hypnotic properties of rose, also that it affects the GABA receptors that govern anxiety and mood, and that rose also affects the memory.

We also recognise PTSD by its symptomatic exaggerated fear responses. You and I also recognise the connections between the kidneys and fear, and also rose's affects on the kidney meridians. Clearly there are still many jigsaw pieces missing. The picture on the outside of the box shows a calmer, less aggressive outcome. I absolutely *promise* you that rose treats PTSD effectively but how that journey exactly takes place, we still do not understand.

Here's what we do know...

Relaxation

We'll start with a very straight forward and clever trial from 2009 where a Japanese researcher with the triumphant name of Hongratanaworakit, and his team, measured physiological indicators of relaxation from rose: **blood pressure, breathing rate, blood oxygen saturation, pulse rate, and skin temperature** were all measured as well as a psychological responses.

The physical feedback showed breathing slowed and both blood oxygen saturation and systolic blood pressures lowered. When their psychological questionnaires were analysed, the rose group were described as calmer, more relaxed and less alert than subjects in the control group

The conclusion of the paper relates: *These findings are likely to represent a relaxing effect of the rose oil and provide some evidence for the use of rose oil in aromatherapy, such as causing relief of depression and stress in humans.*

Hypnotic

In November 2006 it was confirmed that Rosa damascena **affected both the central nervous system** and **the brain** by causing a ***hypnotic quality***. The oil does this **by inhibiting the activity of the hypothalamus and the pituitary gland**. (Here's your HPA axis again)This was assessed by treating rats orally using rose alongside a positive control group who were given diazepam and also a negative control who were treated with saline.

Thirty minutes after their treatments, the rats were then given injections of pentobarbital to slow their brains and their length of time sleeping was recorded. Those that had been treated with an aqueous version of rose experienced longer sleeping times similar to that enjoyed by those that had been treated with diazepam. Those that had been given the chloroformic extract of rose did not experience any hypnotic effects. This means then that our original essential oil, not the chloroformic extract made by the scientists, had the more hypnotic effect on the rats.

http://www.ncbi.nlm.nih.gov/pubmed/17205713

Conflict

When I found this next trial I was deeply involved in finding proof of action on the physical body, and I very nearly discounted it (partly because it was really complex to get my head round and I had an attack of the lazies, but mainly because , my little rats had a horrible time with this one! So prepare yourselves...) when I scrolled down to add it to the emotional dimension notes, it hit me just how very important it was.

It seems to me that the main conditions you would use rose for are depression and anxiety, grief, menopause, PMT and PTSD (seems weird those to abbreviated forms sitting next to each other!) So, what do all of these conditions have in common? I think ***emotional attack mechanism***. How about you?

I am going to skirt around the animal agony a bit because it is quite upsetting and you can always access it for yourself if you have a tougher skin than I.

This is a trial from 1999 where rats were rather cruelly conditioned using electric shocks as a punishment for drinking water. There were several oils assessed (Rose, orange, camomile and ylang ylang) and they were compared with the more scientifically understood, diazepam. With both diazepam and rose, but not the other essential oils, the rats remained undeterred and the poor little things kept going back to try and get a drink. This failure to recognise they need to avoid getting a shock is deemed to be indicative that the creature has been sedated. In other words, he is dopey in the very truest sense of the word.

When trying to ascertain what process the brain was using, the scientists then used an antagonist (effectively an *off switch*) of flumazenil, an injection that reverses the effects of benzodiazepine drugs. In the diazepam rats, this chill pill relaxed the diazepam dopey darlings and they quickly got their s**t together and they wised up to quit trying to drink. But the same did not happen to the rose-tinted rats. Since researchers have an excellent understanding of how flumazenil works, (on the GABA receptors) they were able to verify that this anti-conflict aspect of rose works on a different chemical pathway completely (The understanding of this as yet still remains elusive).

Later in 2000, Umezu et al. built on this knowledge to prove that lavender also has the same anti-conflict properties as rose. Then in 2012 he made a far reaching statement that *"Essential oils of eucalyptus and rose decreased the avoidance rate (number of avoidance responses/number of avoidance trials) without affecting the response rate, indicating that they may exhibit some CNS acting effects. Essential oils of 12 other plants, including juniper, patchouli, geranium, jasmine, clary sage, neroli, lavender, lemon, ylang-ylang, niaouli, vetivert and frankincense had no effect on the avoidance response in mice"*

So, what does that mean for the findings of other essential oils? We'll need to wait with baited breath really, to see what else he has to say. Interesting though, that the two oils you would use if you want to relax but also increase concentration and focus, vetiver and frankincense are both there....no dopey rats in that section then.

1. https://www.aromaticscience.com/anticonflict-effects-of-plant-derived-essential-oils-2/
2. http://www.aromaticscience.com/behavioral-effects-of-plant-derived-essential-oils-in-the-geller-type-conflict-test-in-mice/
3. https://www.aromaticscience.com/evaluation-of-the-effects-of-plant-derived-essential-oils-on-central-nervous-system-function-using-discrete-shuttle-type-conditioned-avoidance-response-in-mice-2/

Memory

Schopolamine is a commonly prescribed drug, which interestingly enough, is plant derived. It is a secondary metabolite from the *Soanaceae* genus, otherwise known as the nightshade family. It is usually given to patients who are suffering some degree of nausea; this might be from vertigo, gastro-intestinal problems including IBS and also travel sickness (where it can be applied as a patch).

There can be side effects of this drug for some people running from dizziness to hallucinations and arrhythmia. (Patients are given a drug that makes them dizzy because they have vertigo and are dizzy?!) Most commonly, people find that it can affect their memory.

On June 29th 2014, (we have to have the full date here because it's my birthday and so that's exciting!) researchers in Iran found that the anti-oxidant effects of *Rosa damascena* were able to affect brain tissues in rats who had been treated with schopolamine, and the rose was seen to prevent the memory deficits doctors might usually expect to see.

You can find this trial here:
http://www.ncbi.nlm.nih.gov/pubmed/24974980

Memory and Alzheimer's

This idea was followed through a little further by researchers in Department of Anatomical Sciences and Molecular Biology, Ifsahan, Iran.

Here they explored the notion that in the early stages of Alzheimer's, the hippocampus is vulnerable in the part it plays in storing memories, but for a time there is some degree of plasticity in the cells. That is to say the neurons in the brain might be replaceable and be able to adapt and repair. Behavioural experiments with rats demonstrated that *Rosa damascena* was able to provoke plasticity leading them to make the suggestion that supplements of *damascena* might serve as a preventative in the fight against Alzheimer's, and could possibly ameliorate the effects of mild memory problems.

This abstract to this trial can be found at http://www.ncbi.nlm.nih.gov/pubmed/24395280

Anxiety

A proper bit of aromatherapy for a change instead of all this rose extract malarkey. This is inhalation of rose essential oil versus oral administration in rats. Here three groups were analysed, a control group, a group with induced Chronic Mild Stress and two rose groups, one with oral administration and one via inhalation.

So the rodent regime was for 28 days and at the end, cerebral cortex samples were taken from the group (Read fast and maybe the full impact of the last sentence might not register!)

On analysis levels of vitamin A, vitamin E, vitamin C and β-carotene were all lower in the control group than the stressed group, but they were *higher* in one of the rose oil groups. Interestingly the changes had not taken place in the oral administration group, only the vapour trialled. Likewise the lipids in the blood had oxidised significantly in the control group, more so in the CNS group, but the levels were decreased in the rose inhalation group.

The paper makes the leap then of saying that depression seems to be caused by oxidative stress and that inhalation of *Rosa damascena* protects against this oxidative deterioration.

Want some ammunition against the advocates of random essential oil ingestion? Why not start with this trial http://www.ncbi.nlm.nih.gov/pubmed/22484603

A very quick hat tip to a very straightforward trial from 2004 where rats were treated to varying doses of rose oil by inhalation (1.0%, 2.5%, and 5.0%) and then were sent into maze to see how stressed they were. At all doses the rats were entirely comfortable scurrying around the maze and exploring, as opposed to their usual response of finding a dark corner to hide in. 1% then, people, I do like it when I can give you proof to keep your essential oil expenditure down!!!

Anxiety and withdrawal

I said before that one of the teams involved in the male sexuality trial was mainly interested in substance abuse. This theme arises several times throughout the research I have found with rose. This time, the study looks specifically at morphine withdrawal and the way that rose affects the GABA receptors.

A quick physiology recap for you: GABA receptors (Gamma Aminobutyric Acid). These neurotransmitters are some of the most important aspects of our chemical nervous system. They are responsible for excitability of the nervous system but also the regulation of smooth muscle.

Here the essential oil was injected inter peritoneally (into their tummies), and the effects of the rose were compared, firstly with a placebo control and then also a group of rats which had been administered with diazepam

Both rose and diazepam reduced the number of jumping episodes the rats had.

Both also decreased the “wet dog shake”. As the dilution was increased more improvements started to occur. At both dilutions of 5% and 20% rooming, climbing and writhing all started to improve.

When the dilution reached a massive 40%, the rats stopped rearing up and their teeth chattering diminished too.

The only one disappointing thing was that rose seemed to have no effect on the diarrhoea that the withdrawal caused.

In every case, except for the diarrhoea, the rose brought about similar relief to the animal addicts as diazepam had done. The only one area that diazepam did hold the upper hand was this diarrhoea issue where it had reduced symptoms but rose had not.

So then, I wonder how this wonder medicine was reducing the agony of those poor withdrawing rats. Researchers seem more than happy that it affects the GABA receptors somehow, but as yet, they do not understand *in which way*.

To quote the authors of the study: "*In conclusion it seems that GABAergic activity induced by flavonoids from Rosa damascena essential oil can alleviate signs of morphine withdrawal, but further studies need to be done to better understand this mechanism.*"

Chapter 10 The Spiritual dimension of rose

The Chakras

There will be no surprises about the subtle healing of rose. It balances the heart chakra and also the crown. These energy centres connect the etheric bodies of the aura with the physical body. In health they rotate open and closed vitalising the organs of the body. They can however jam open or closed restricting or overpowering the organs with emotions that don't serve us well.

The heart chakra is located, as one would imagine in the centre of the chest. It is governed by our capacity to love and to be loved. Emotions like grief of anger affect the heart chakra which is then translated into the physical body. Here we see problems in the chest, so lung and heart problems specifically. The best demonstration of this energy would be love, but also grief.

The crown chakra is more complex in that it connects us with the outer universe. It is the seat of cosmic connection, it is from here we develop compassion and empathy, but likewise we might see problems with the head and with the brain. For this power region we would hope for peace, but in the same way we can see its opposite number of war....Innana power.

The science of Vibration

Everything in the universe has a vibration. If you cast your mind back to school, you might recall learning how molecules are always constantly vibrating against each other. Those molecules closest together maintain a solid state, further apart makes things more fluid and so they have a liquid state and the most disparate molecules take the form of a vapour or gas. The reason we have solids, liquids and gas is because of vibration and we call this vibration... **energy.**

Everything in life has a speed of vibration. The more pure something is, the higher its vibration is. In the same way if there is some degree of pollution then the vibration is dragged down too. In the late 1990's a biophysicist by the name of Bruce Tainio invented a machine called the BT3 Monitor that measured the vibrations of plants. His findings have become the stuff of urban legend and Tainio's name seems synonymously linked with Gary Young of Young Living Oils. I can't decide how I feel about that. I don't *think* it compromises the quality of *this* work per se.

Essential oils are said to have produced the highest of all the frequencies given off in his machine, with rose soaring way above every other with a frequency of 320Hz. Production of the BT3 monitor has been discontinued, but there are many other metaphysical arts that do back up the findings of the monitor.

- The brain of a genius resonates between 83mhz to 98Hz

- The standard healthy body and mind is said to be vibrate at somewhere between76mhz to 83mhz

- Colds, flu and illness drag the vibration down to 57mhz to 63mhz

- Cancer receptors vibrate at 42mhz

The ideal then, is to find a way to raise our vibration in order to lift us above the illness resonance. Research backs up the idea that meditation and prayer do this.

Feeling happy does this and laughter too. If the research is to be believed plant and crystal medicines are some of the most effective ways of doing this.

(My problem with the YL issue is we now have this marketing spin that if you swallow an essential oil then we immediately become purer and that, I am afraid ladies and gentlemen, is utter rubbish. A bad person who drinks anything is still a bad person! Swallowing something is not going to change that!)

Plants always work on three levels - mind, body & spirit. Usually though, you find properties are very heavily weighted towards one or two rather than all three. I feel this is so with rose, in that it has very physical and spiritual dimensions, but less so for the mental aspects. It almost seems like the mental dimension is like a child being lead along on a leash! This is probably because one of the foremost properties of the medicine is that it ensures that **the head always listens to the heart.**

What's more rose is a **soul medicine,** probably even more than it pertains to the spirit. If that is an alien sentence to you, consider that the soul has many incarnations but the spirit has only one. The spirit is very much **the essence of you**, however the soul pathway is far more about the accumulated knowledge you have gained through *many* incarnations.

I think this is a valuable thing to consider because it helps you to access those innate abilities that have been brought with you into this life from previous ones. It also helps you to grasp traumas that are travelling through time with you too. Potentially their original trauma belonged to another being entirely, and yet their physical effects may plague you still.

Consider the soul pathway to be an endless line.

Birth and death are merely knots in the thread, but the string continues onwards, collecting data (both good and bad) and taking it from one life to the next. Rose is extremely good at following that thread. It helps you access talents and skills that come easily to you. It helps you to make sense of why they might be important, but it also dissipates trauma from long ago.

The healing energy of rose is to remind you *why* you are here and to demonstrate to you just how rich your

gifts are. The medicine is very clever at accessing residual memories that have set up patterns of behaviour. It allows you to reset their imprint.

Often it can be tempting to shut out painful memories because the agony can be just too acute.

Courage mon brave...

Because inside that shell of discomfort lies the pearl of wisdom you were sent here to learn.

Do you remember that old Heineken advert "Refreshes the parts that other beers can't reach" Here, I think you can replace Heineken for rose. Its gentle healing permeates through the skin to the very soul, travels through this incarnation to traumas from many generations before. Truly, rose must be a gateway to God.

Jill Bruce describes Rose Otto in her book The Garden of Eden:

Allows one to feel and understand the presence of God. Used by people with a spiritual link to the Almighty.

This oil can be used to bring about many kinds of healing. Its properties seem to be enhanced by the purity of the healer. It has a capacity to blend with human consciousness and magnify its own healing capacities. One drop mixed with other oils will also magnify their healing abilities. It seems to add divine energy.

Chapter 11 The Magick of the Rose

Archetype

Archetypes are patterns found in universal consciousness. That is, we recognise their story regardless of our religion or social background. Consider Mary, Mother of God as wholesome and innocent, versus the temptation of the snake in the Garden of Eden. Of Father Christmas versus the Grinch, they are stories that elicit deep recognitions in our psyche. The eminent psychologists Carl Jung described archetypes as being part of our collective unconsciousness and as such are part of the imagery of art, dreams and religions. I find these myths very helpful understanding the complete dynamic of a plant.

The Myth of Isis

One could choose Aphrodite, Venus or Innana, but I think the most complete aspect of rose is depicted in the archetype of Isis.

Again some of the earliest wisdom we have to draw on about her comes from Plutarch (he, who also bought us the Cleopatra in the gilded boat story) in his poem *De Iside et Osiride.*

Here he describes how Isis was the daughter of Nut and Geb, the sky god and goddess of night. One of five children, Isis was to become entangled in one of the strangest sibling/lover relationships ever seen in history. Betrothed to her brother husband Osiris, Isis became consort to a beloved, powerful and inspiring king. Jealous of Osiris' power, their brother Set began a fearful plot to kill him.

Throwing an elaborate banquet for Osiris, Set brought with him a magnificently ornate box and declared everyone in the kingdom must try it out for size. Osiris, playing along, lay inside it, discovering that he fitted it perfectly. Unbeknownst to Osiris, his scheming brother had secretly measured him as he slept, so when the heavy lid came down with a fearful crash, it fastened itself firmly shut. Set, gleeful at the success of his plan despatched the box gently into the Nile. .

For many days the coffin ebbed and flowed, gently moving further away from Isis with the tide. It seemed to travel endlessly until suddenly, with great force, it hit a cedar tree and became completely entrenched in the trunk. Meanwhile, back at the palace, Isis was distraught.

She lamented her beloved husband, in anguish for the destiny of his soul. How could he reach the Land of The Dead, she wondered, without a proper burial? Isis was filled with purpose and righteous indignation and set off on a journey to bring the body of her beloved Osiris back to her. Changing herself into a bird, she set off across the world to find her lover. After many months of searching she found the beautiful box that contained her one true love.

Taking it home she concealed the coffin for fear of Set discovering it. Furious, Set searched for and found the box then cut Osiris into 14 different parts casting them to all four corners of the world.

Poor Isis was desolate but she would not be beaten. Recruiting Set's sister wife Nephthys, together they scoured every inch of the land. One by one, Isis was able to recover the pieces that remained of Osiris. Still missing his phallus, because a fish had devoured his final part, Isis was able to recover 13 of the 14 pieces. Isis, a great sorceress, set about reconstructing her love, forming a giant golden phallus to complete her masterpiece. With the help of Thoth she reattached it to Osiris and then danced a fearsome ritual around the body, chanting the dismembered Osiris back to life.

Then, transforming herself once more, she took on the form of a bird, this time a kite, hovered over the body and magically conceived a son with Osiris, Horus. Peacefully Osiris was despatched to the underworld.

The medicine of the myth

Perhaps, different from other plants where we seek *truths* from the myths, the rose *is* the embodiment of Isis. Through her fragrance we are connected with the feminine divine.

Isis, the daughter of the god of day and the goddess of night, is in the very truest sense about wholeness. Unlike other nature goddesses she has a shadow side that she is not afraid to embrace. She will conjure, trick and seduce and this is the very root of her power.

She recognises that her magic is not complete without the masculine element and she needs to embrace that to bring Osiris back to life. Her power is so extraordinary that it can overcome death, but it requires sexual union to achieve this.

There is medicine from Isis, because she understands the feeling of having part of you taken away and she recognises that moving towards death without healing this aspect cannot be good.

She finds a way to heal grief, by communicating in a way that even death cannot compromise.

This is the first time we hear of how majestic the might of Isis is. It is **her anger and great wrath that galvanises her power.** It is what brings her, her sense of purpose. But over and above the fury she feels at Set is the compassion she feels for her husband. It is the knowing that he should have a good burial that gives her the drive to carry on. It is the openness of her heart that drives her ever onward.

And then of course, we have this desire she has to procreate; for Osiris to have a legacy, and the magic she performs to achieve that. The magic of a goddess cradled in the potency of rose.

Ruling Planet

Venus

In astrology Venus represents, not only love, but also money. More it represents how we feel about these things. She governs our sentiments about *pleasure,* our values in life, our artistic and creative endeavours and our tastes.

Venus is sociable, attractive and delicious! She mingles and always lights up the room. She is erudite and expressive. She is passionate and more than just a little bit sexy!

Element

Air

Plants that fall under the Greek element of air pertain to their mental capacities. They are aloof and detached, they are cool and artistic.

In balance, air energy is kind, intellectual, communicative and social. Out of balance the energy turns selfish, superficial, and vicious. Stagnant or deficient air energy is insensitive to other people's emotions.

Sacred Geometry

What's interesting to perceive about the rose is how its form fits into sacred geometry. The placement of the petals, arranged like a pentagram unfold to the pattern of Fibonacci sequence.

1, 1, 2, 3, 5, 13, 18,

Each layer of petals has more, but the number is not accidental. The spiral of petals increases by 1.618 each cycle, the number of the Golden Ratio. Centuries of study have demonstrated that this golden ratio forms the geometry of images that are the most appealing to the eye. It shows itself in the distances between features in our most beautiful people, in some of the world's most impressive structures and in enigmatic music too. It is most famously illustrated in Da Vinci's painting Vitruvian Man. Can you see how the lines and spirals dissect the image? This golden ratio is the same in the geometry of the rose.

Fascinatingly we see it show itself in nature over and over again. Yes, in the rose, but also the sunflower, the seashell and the fern are just a few examples that come to mind. Whirlwinds spiral, waves curl and break and even plants orbit around the earth in this ratio. (Funnily enough it takes Venus 1.6 years to circle the earth!) This has led many people suggest that the golden ratio is more than simply maths, but in fact the divine proportion of God – that the Golden ratio is the extender of the most divine energy.

Most certainly I find this to be true of the healing energy of rose.

It is timeless, boundless and limitless. It has the ability to cross lifetimes and bring about healing mechanisms that science can only dream of

Memories and traumas can melt through lifetimes and rose is able to access them in a way that no steel surgical tool has the capacity to do. Perhaps, this is a past lives issue, but it is also a ***homeopathic*** one too.

One of the main concepts of homeopathy is miasm, **the inherited predisposition of a disease**. This is a massive book in its own right, but it is one way to explain why certain families are more predisposed to certain illnesses. There are several different miasms which contain various different ailments and they are believed to be derived from an ancient trauma in the ancestor's DNA. According to homeopathy, problems in a family such as alcoholism, insanity and heart disease may be attributed to a horrible infection contracted many generations ago

The syphilitic miasm trespassed into a bloodline when mother contracted syphilis during pregnancy and her child's health became severely compromised. As the generations pass, each person carries with them some throwback from the attack. Even a century later the syphilitic throwback can be seen. Making up about 15% of all diseases, we see syphilitic miasm presenting as diseases of the nervous system, the blood and skeleton. Psychological disorders such as alcoholism, depression, suicidal impulses and insanity prevail. You might also see a loss of smell and taste, blindness, deafness and ulcerations. It is also associated with many heart conditions, some vesicular skin eruptions and diseases that seem to only show themselves at night (restless legs, insomnia, nightmares etc...).

Now if you find nothing else strange in this book, an inherited disposition towards certain illnesses and emotional issues should certainly give you pause especially when I tell you one of the oils to cut the thread of syphilitic miasm is rose.

Often rose is used as an essence (and here I refer to the vibrational flower water as opposed to the essential oil) Their best effects are found in emotional healing for treating sadness, depression, addiction, obsessions and self harming. All of these dreadful mechanisms we use as self hatred in this human condition, resultant from denying our feelings, pushing them down and hiding them.

Traumas of any physical, emotional or spiritual source can have the same effect on us, that we divorce ourselves from our heart. We close ourselves down to protect us from any further pain. We recoil. We put up barriers....

We develop thorns.

Maybe the trauma belongs to this lifetime and experience, or perhaps another. These traumas do not even need to be separated by a *physical* death either. My biggest trauma belongs to a whole different me; the one who lived with a man who beat and shamed me at every opportunity. *That* me doesn't even exist anymore but neither was she cremated or buried. She and I share a skin, but nothing more. (And actually I can thank rose for how easily I shed that skin and formed a new beautiful one. A psychological skin and a rather lovely facial complexion too!)

Rose Vibration

Music

Just as all things have a vibration then some of these things overlap. In the same way the symbolism of a red rose has very deeply understood meaning, the healing properties of a rose don't necessarily have to come from an oil. Sometimes they can some from imagery and music too.

So then, to summon up the power of rose we *can* sit cross legged and breathe in its scent floating on cosmic rays, or we can tune into the vibration in other ways too.

My personal channel is through music, because I hear essential oils as musical notes. This is very useful to me because it means that any music I play has to be in absolute accord with the vibrations of the oils I choose. It also helps me when I am blending oils because if I choose an oil that jars it sounds like the cat is walking over the piano!

The vibration of rose is a clear resounding C. It chimes rich and strong like a bell. C Major is probably the first scale we all learned on the piano, from middle C by the screws marking the middle of the keyboard up to the next C. It is that second C that is the sound of rose. It is commonly accepted that keys have their own personalities and Bob Dylan is quoted as describing C major as "the key of strength, but also the key of regret".

I collated this list on a Saturday morning in the living room. Toy Story 3 was on the TV, the handsome man was cooking bacon in the kitchen. I had my headphones on and I sat quietly with tears streaming down my face. The man just came in, shook his head and laughed at me. But play the list and you will see why I was marvelling and weeping. The following are all songs written in that same key of C whose souls, I feel, demonstrate the healing energies of rose.

Cleverly C chimes out the opening bars of **Bette Midler's** hauntingly hopeful song about love, called **The Rose**.

The call to compassionate arms of **John Lennon's Imagine** entirely encompasses this joining of heart and crown chakra energies. Pure rose peace, and I love the idea that the rose seems to transcend the barrier that has brought most wars "And no religion too". Innana, Aphrodite, Venus, Mary...

The Beatles summon up rose energy through incantations to Mother Mary in **Let It Be**. Rose energy...written in C

I'll lay the gauntlet down to listen to **James Morrison's Broken Strings** and not see rose prescriptions in every single line.

My all time favourite piece of music **Private Investigations,** by **Dire Straits** might seem not to fit but that lonely man sitting in his smoke filled dingy office, nursing his whiskey and pain behind his eyes....jaded, cynical and worn out with life. Yes, that's entirely rose prescription.

(I think since we are looking to learn rose medicine through music, it would be remiss of me not to mention **Kelly Clarkson's** ***Because of You*** even though it is written in G Minor. That level of anger and distrust would certainly warrant rose.)

The agony of rose medicine sings through the lyrics of all these songs. But rose energy is birth, life, death, *rebirth*...there is always a pink ray of hope that begins very faintly but soon begins to grow and flood the heart with a more positive outlook.

Air supply's *All out of Love* laments

" I wish I could carry your smile in my heart

For times when my life seems so low

It would make me believe what tomorrow could bring

When today doesn't really know, doesn't really know"

Waiting for the spring...

And as those early buds of May start to show, the pain is not so acute then **Kelly Clarkson** hammers out another anthem that I reckon every teenage kid should be taught in school...What doesn't kill ya makes you **stronger**. "Thanks to you I'm finally thinking about me... Just me, myself and I"

That thread of dependency finally breaks....the liberation of independence at last. Take a deep breath and fill those lungs with all the space left now that pain in your chest has gone

But rose isn't all about pain...it's even more about hope. Hope for tomorrow, but also hope of finding out just how powerful you can be. Finding that elusive reason why the universe needs you, and absolutely no-one else will do.

Cyndi Lauper's True Colours begins

"You with the sad eyes

Don't be discouraged

Oh I realize

It's hard to take courage

In a world full of people

You can lose sight of it all

And the darkness inside you

Can make you feel so small

This song positively drips rose essence, from the sadness and confidence aspects to the belief that "*your true colours are beautiful like a rainbow.*"

Want to capture those rose scented sunshine in the garden moments? Get in the car, whack the top down and feel the wind in your hair....Now play **Daft Punk's Fragments of Time** as loud as you can. You can almost smell dog roses wafting in the air.

Ok, are ya ready to party it out? After all rose essence raises our vibration but so does laughter and I heartily believe in the power of dance. Let's see those hips samba rolling to **Phil Collin's Dance into the Light**. How about of a bit of Venus energy with **Madonna's Material Girl** or perhaps **John Paul Young's Love is in The Air**...

Remember what you think most about is what you attract....

But the finale though, must always end with a diva, and no-one even comes close to belting out that glorious anthem of hope, **One Moment in Time by Whitney Houston.**

Grab your hairbrushes ladies...I wanna hear you sing out loud and proud!

I want one moment in time

When I'm more than I thought I could be

When all of my dreams are a heartbeat away

And the answers are all up to me

Give me one moment in time

When I'm racing with destiny

Then in that one moment of time

I will feel

I will feel eternity

Timeless rose medicine...For Goddess sake...let's have some hope.

Imagery

In a quieter, more refined space, we find a contemplative healing of a different kind. I'd like to introduce you to the healing effects of channelling rose imagery.

Pioneered by Sandy Humby, Rose Alchemy is the most beautiful set of rose cards. Each card carries a different medicine transported through the photograph of the plant on the card into the energetic medicine using meditation and intention.

Every picture has been taken by Sandy herself as she has travelled the planet learning the secrets of the rose. Within each image is the energy that can be summoned from the rose.

Sandy described to me how, if the soul has not healed before it leaves the body, then it becomes stuck. From there the body takes on the energetic imprint of the trauma and carries it through the soul journey. Marvellously, when she is healing she is able to actually able to see threads hanging from the rear of the heart chakra. From there she is able to tug on them in and trace back to where the story of the pain began.

She takes the imagery of her rose images, choosing the most appropriate one and then she plants the mental image into the organ to realign the body's blue print. The rose energy remains there, pulsating and revitalising the organ, until it is ready to send its energy to the heart to enable it to open again.

The wisdom of these roses was originally given to her during meditation. When she received them, she was told she was being given the roses to heal The Magdalena Wound. I find this fascinating. Looking at the ancient goddesses that have walked with rose, the age of feminine emancipation seems to be taking us back to the idea of men and women as co-creators with their deity. That the endless guilt women have carried for their connection with their sexuality is at an end. In 1969 the Catholic Church admitted that there *had* never been any grounds for calling the Magdalena "whore". As society begins to assimilate women back into their wholeness of sexual, powerful beings so the rose follows Her goddess energy still.

I must take this opportunity to thank Sandy not only for the use of her images but the depth of knowledge that she added to the symbolic aspects of the book, in particular the Golden Ratio work.

Chapter 12 Traditional Medicine Recipes

How to make a Flower Essence

You may have come across Bach Flower Remedies, or similar flower essences. They are a beautiful way of conveying the vibrational healing of a plant....and a good site cheaper than essential oils!

Find yourself a beautiful glass bowl and set it aside for making flower essences and nothing else.

You will need some water. The best possible scenario is that it has been flowing close to where your plant has been growing. That might not always be possible, so it is fine to buy spring water, however tap water tends to have too much fluoride added. .

A funnel

A dark glass bottle (125ml is a good size).

Alcohol (at least 40%, such as vodka).

Directions

So, before we do any picking, it is nice to just tune into the flower and thank it for the medicine you are about to take. Strangely sometimes you might have a sense that suddenly that flower does not feel right. Follow your intuition and choose another one the same way until you find one you like.

Fill your bowl with spring water and place it amongst the flowers you are collecting, and allow it to warm and charge from the sun.

We always make flower essences on sunny days. This allows the sun's rays to help transmit the healing message through the petals in to the water. This is process is called solarisation.

Be very aware of avoiding imprinting too much on the essence. When we are making an essential oil remedy, it helps to purposely charge the blend with love, but in vibrational essences, clearly we want to harness the healing energies of the *plant*. Drop the petals onto the surface of the water, covering its surface, but then leave them alone. (If you stir it, you are making an infusion, not an essence.) Ensure it is in a bright spot, where no shadows can impede the solarisation, then find something else to do for two hours.

When we come back to the bowl, we are going to want to remove the flowers. No fingers or metal please. Sticks or wooden spoons work best. Do not touch the water because again, we don't want your imprint, we want the rose vibration.

Decant into the bottle to the halfway mark then top up with alcohol.

We call this the "**mother essence**" we use this to fill our treatment bottles, which are usually 20ml (1oz) with little pipette droppers.

Use only seven drops from the Mother Essence and fill the rest with alcohol to make your treatment.

Dosages

Take a couple of drops in water, or directly under the tongue, as often as you think about it, preferably as far away from meals as possible.

Because the action is very subtle, it easy to start the treatment but then to forget to carry on with the regime. Try to carry on for 21 days if you can.

The 17th Century herbalist Culpepper gives us some excellent instructions about how to use the roses we find in the garden. He extols the virtues of the Damask Rose and states that only this and the Dog Rose have medical properties.

The flowers of the common red rose dried, are given in infusions, and sometimes in powder, against overflowings of the menses, spitting of blood, and other hæmorrhages. There is likewise an elegant tincture made from them by pouring a pint of boiling water on half an ounce of the dried petals, and adding fifteen drops of the oil of vitriol and three or four drachms of the finest sugar in powder, after which they are to be stirred together, and left to cool leisurely. This tincture, when poured clear off, is of a beautiful red colour. It may be taken to the amount of three or spoonfuls, twice or three times a day, for strengthening the stomach, and preventing vomiting. It is likewise a powerful and pleasant remedy in immoderate discharges of the menses, and all other fluxes and hæmorrhages. Culpepper

How to make Tinctures

Tinctures are popular ways to take herbal medicine because they have a very long shelf life and can be easily carried around in your pocket. Great, if you need to be taking your medicine frequently, tinctures preserve the plant matter in alcohol. Vodka is usually the liquor of choice but as long as it is tasteless and is more than 80% proof, the choice is yours.

Find a glass or ceramic container with a lid. Avoid metal as it reacts with the alcohol and changes the properties of the blend.

The ratio of herbs to alcohol varies dependant on whether they are dried or fresh.

Use as follows:

1. Add enough fresh chopped herbs to fill the glass container. Cover with alcohol

OR

2. Add 4 ounces (113g) of powdered herb with 1 pint (473ml) of alcohol (or vinegar/glycerine)

OR

3. Add 7 ounces (198g) of dried herb material to 35 fluid ounces (1 litre) of alcohol (or vinegar/glycerine).

Stir round with a blunt knife ensuring all air pockets are dispersed.

Seal the lid well and place in a dark, cool place for 2 weeks, shaking regularly.

When the time has elapsed, take a piece of muslin or a tea towel to catch all the plant matter and allow the liquid to seep through into a bowl below. Squeeze gently.

Decant the tincture into a small dark glass bottle and seal well. Label clearly and keep out reach of children.

Kept properly, a tincture has a shelf life of around five years.

How to make Infusions

Infusions are remedies which are drunk, much like a cup of tea. 2 tablespoons of plant matter is placed in a jar, covered with boiling water and left to steep with a lid on, for between 4-6 hours. This might be a good way to enjoy a homemade rose petal tea. You might decide to make infusions of hips which is very similar to how they are used in TCM, or you might want to make a gentle treatment to cool sunburn etc....

How to make Decoctions

Unlike infusions, decoctions use rigorous boiling as a means to extract the properties from more stubborn matter such as woods and spices. This would definitely be more suited to hips than to petals, but experiment and find your own way.

Use a heavy pan and around 2 tablespoons of plant matter to 1 cup of water. Bring to a boil and then simmer for around 20 minutes.

Decant and allow to cool to drinking temperature before use.

How to Make Macerations

This is one of my personal favourite ways to "capture the magic of the garden". Clearly a maceration is not going to be as strong as an essential oil, but it makes wonderful carrier oil. I usually make my macerations with sunflower oil but if you follow Ayurvedic and Ancient Egyptian principles than sesame might work better.

Fill a bottle or jar with the vegetable oil, any oil will do. Fill it full of plant matter, petals, herbs or spices and ensure they are completely covered with the oil. Leave it for a month on the windowsill in the sunshine. The vegetable oil takes the essential oils of the plant into it and you have a lovely magical oil.

In the immortal words of Robert Herrick:

Gather your rosebuds, while ye may...

For time is surely flying."

How to make a Poultice

A poultice is often more recently referred to as a compress. It is used to place herbs or oils onto the skin to either draw out toxin and poisons or to allow the herbs to sit atop a wound for quickest healing. Poultices can either be warm (to open the pores) or cold (to shut them down again). By alternating warm and cold, opening and closing the pores repeatedly, toxicity is drawn to the surface. This is useful in cases of abscesses or even nasty blemishes for example.

Soak a cloth in water, add the herbs and place over the wound. It can help to bandage the herbs in place. To add essential oils, add 3 drops to the water before soaking. Try to use extreme temperatures which are still comfortable, so the hottest or coldest you can bear. Always test the water for temperature to avoid scalding.

Cold compresses for sunburn, temperatures or scalding

Warm compresses just because your skin will positively adore you for it!!

How to Make Rosehip syrup

Often tinctures and decoctions can be unpalatable to children. A syrup is the answer as it is sweet and comforting.

"This syrup is an excellent purge for children, and there is not a better medicine for grown people of a costive habit, for a small quantity of it taken every night will keep the bowels soluble, and constantly open." Culpepper

During World War II the Ministry of Defence issued recipes for rosehip syrup to every household in Britain. The mega dose of vitamin C was a welcome herald ready for the cold winters that lay ahead.

900g (2 lbs) of rosehips

2.5ltrs (4.5 pts) water

450 g (1lb) white granulated sugar

Method:

- Bring 1½ litres (3 pts) of water to the boil.

- Mince the rosehips through your food processor. Chuck them is as they are. No need to top and tail because they will be strained later.

- Carefully pour the fruit into the boiling water and wait until it comes back to the boil. Remove your pan from the heat and leave the hips to steep for about 15 minutes.

- Pour through a sterilised jelly bag/or muslin square and let as much of syrup drip through as you can

- Return the pulp to your pan and add 1.5 pts of fresh boiling water. Bring it to the boil again. Remove from heat and leave for 15 minutes infuse again.

- Repeat the straining again.

- Now, pour all your syrup into a clean saucepan, bring it to the boil again, simmer and reduce to 1.5 pts / 1litre.

- Add the sugar and boil your mixture rapidly for a final 5 minutes. Pour into hot sterile bottles and seal immediately.
- To test consistency, drip a droplet of the syrup into a glass of cold water. If it splits into pieces, boil a little longer.
- If the drop remains intact, the syrup is ready to bottle into a sterilized container.

How to sterilize jars and bottles

Use only glass containers for herbal medicines. Wash with warm soapy water and rinse well. Do not towel dry. Place face down onto the rack shelves of a preheated oven at 150 degrees Fahrenheit /65 degrees Celsius and leave for 20 minutes.

Meanwhile boil the lids for 5 minutes.

Always heat your bottles to meet the temperature of your liquid to avoid cracking.

How to Make Rose sugar

Take equal parts of rose petals and sugar.

Chopped the white end off each rose petal because this tastes bitter

Fine chop the rose petals

Place some sugar into a pestle and mortar and pound the petals into the sugar.

Use the sugar immediately if you want it to be this pretty pink. Otherwise store in an airtight container where it will keep for about six months. The next day though, the petals will have turned brown. This still works beautifully mixed into cakes though, and rather than that ethereal rosy scent it changes to more rosehip fruity note.

This is beautiful for baking with, or adding to a lovely cup of very refined tea.

Most impressive though...dip a cocktail glass into egg white and then into rose sugar...

Now that ladies and gentlemen really *is* cosmopolitan!

Rose Petal Congee

Many thanks to kaleidecope.cultural-china.com for the following anti-aging rose petal recipe:

Put in a pot 80g of short grain rice, 15g of wolfberry fruit, 10 red dates and 15g of sesame seeds. Simmer them on low heat until the mixture reaches a boil, and then drop in 10g of dried rose petals.

Now I gotta tell ya.... Rose petal congee *really* didn't float my boat, but this recipe for rose petal porridge really put wind in my sails!

Rose Petal Porridge

Serves 1

- 4 cardamom pods
- 70g (2 ½ oz) porridge oats
- 200ml (7 fl oz) coconut milk
- 1 teaspoon rosewater or 4 drops edible rose essential oil
- 2 tablespoons crushed pistachio nuts
- Maple syrup to serve (optional)
- crystallized rose petals, to decorate (optional)

Crush the cardamom pods with the back of a spoon and drop them into the coconut milk. Bring to the boil and turn down to simmer

Add the oats and gently cook for about 8 minutes

Stir the blend well to prevent sticking and to agitate the seeds.

When the oats are nicely soft take off the heat.

Stir in the rosewater or essential oil, and mix it in well.

Pour in a serving bowl and top with the crushed pistachios, a drizzle of maple syrup and crystallized rose petals, if you want to go the extra mile!

How to Make Rose Petal Jam

There is a conserve made of the unripe flowers, which has nearly the same properties as the syrup; there is likewise a conserve made with the fruit of the wild or dog rose, which is

very pleasant, and of considerable efficacy for common colds and coughs: Culpeper

500g (1lb) fresh rose petals

500g (1lb) white granulated sugar

1 litre (35 fl oz)of water

Juice of 2 lemons

- Identify the most fragrant roses in the garden. Make sure your roses are pesticide and chemical free.
- The jam will take on the hue of your blooms so choose a single colour way of blossoms, all red, all pink etc. Watch for the roses to bloom and cut the heads just before they reach their most glorious fullness.
- Sort through your rose petals and find the beautiful ones. Choose ones that are vibrant with health, fresh and robust. Ensure you wash all petals thoroughly to remove any dirt or tiny insects

- Spread the rose petals in a bowl then sprinkle a drizzle of the sugar over them. Make sure every petal is coated well with sugar. Gently bruise the petals with your fingers as you carefully blend them together with the sugar.

- Cover the bowl tightly with cling film and place it into a refrigerator overnight so that scent of the rose petals has chance to really infuse into the sugar.

Day 2

- Place a small plate into the freezer to chill

- Pour the rest of the sugar into a saucepan with the water and lemon juice.

- Gently heat the contents, stirring all the time.

- Just before the mixture reaches boiling point, carefully add the rose petal and sugar mixture. It is important to keep stirring all the time. Ensure no petals are left resting on the bottom of the pan

- Maintain a steady simmer for around 20 minutes, regularly checking and stirring.

- Now bring the saucepan to a good rolling boil. After around 5 to 10 minutes or so you will see the mixture start to thicken.
- Remove the cold plate from the freezer and drop a small amount of the jam onto it.
- If the jam retains its shape, it is ready. Give it a gentle poke to ensure it has gone solid.
- Let the jam cool a little in the pan. After about 15 minutes pour into sterilised jars.
- When completely cool, cover with waxed discs and put the tops on.
- Label with the date. Jars will last 4 months if kept unopened in the refrigerator

Chapter 13 Essential Oil Recipes

Dry Skin

100mls (4oz) Blank Moisturiser

Rose x 1

Geranium x 1

Cardamom x 1

Sensitive Skin

100mls (4oz) Blank Moisturiser

Rose x1

Melissa x 1

Camomile x 1

Moisturiser to rejuvenate skin after stress

100mls (4oz) Blank Moisturiser

Rose x1

Holy Basil x1

Frankincense x2

Moisturiser to replenish the skin after illness

100mls (4oz) Blank Moisturiser

2 tsp camellia Carrier Oil

2 tsp rosehip carrier oil

1 tsp wheat germ oil

Rose x 1

Vetiver x 1

Cardamom x 1

My favourite spa scrub!

I am a bit of a steam room and sauna junkie, because it helps my lungs so much, so I have a genuine excuse for skiving off work to chill in the Jacuzzi, which is über cool. It would be pretty lax of me to skimp on the products so I have been experimenting with scrubs to help with the detoxification process. This one is formula 27(oh yes Mr, Taxman, Sir, that is how many times I need to go to perfect a formula, and it will say so on my Tax return, but something tells me I might have to have to smile incredibly sweetly to get away with that one...!) and to my mind, it is the final word on relaxation bless and deliciously clean skin.

100g 4oz sea salt

25g 1oz crushed rose petals

25g 1oz frankincense resin

1tsp rosehip carrier oil

1 tbs borage carrier oil

Rose x 1

Vetiver x 1

Cypress x 1

Spa Cream

This is what I use to nourish and condition the skin and lock in the moisture of the oils

100ml 4ox blank moisturiser

1 tsp calendula

1 x vetiver

1 x patchouli

1 x rose

Support for the Hypothalamus (useful in PTSD)

100ml (4oz) Evening Primrose Oil

Rose x 1

Vetiver x 1

Celery seed x 1

Massage into the shoulder mantle and the back of the neck

Memory Problems

Perhaps might be useful in dementia

Rose x 1

Melissa x 1

Lavender x 1

Drop into warm water and make a lovely warm flannel to wash the patient's face.

Eyes

25ml (1 oz) Rosewater

Camomile matricaria x 1

Angelica x 1

Make cooling compresses for the eyes

Digestion

I know I am a beggar for repetition, but I think that it bears reiteration that 90% of the mood modulator serotonin is found in the gut. There is a very strong connection between stress and digestion problems. I don't think it is accidental that we call them tummy upsets! So here we use rose for its digestive properties but also for its calming abilities too.

Massage into the abdomen in a clockwise motion; up the right hand side of your tummy twice, above your belly button twice, down the left hand side twice, and below your belly button just once (so you don't over stimulate the bladder). Use five times a day, just enough oil to make your hand slide is enough.

3 tbs coconut oil

1tsp sesame oil

Rose x 1

Cardamom x 2

Coriander x 3

Ginger x 2

Sexual Dysfunction

For both men and women. Use 2-3 times daily, rubbing into the abdomen and lower back.

Rose x 1

Jasmine x 1

Nutmeg x 1

Damiana x1

Sandalwood x 1

Aphrodisiac

Not every essential oil preparation has to be able illness and dysfunction...!Add some rosy warmth to your loving embrace

2tbs almond oil

1tsp sesame oil

Rose x1

Orange x2

Sandalwood x2

Period pains

Massage into the abdomen in a clockwise motion; up the right hand side of your tummy twice, above your belly button twice, down the left hand side twice, and below your belly button just once (so you don't over stimulate the bladder). Use five times a day, just enough oil to make your hand slide is enough.

Use once a day throughout your cycle. Incidentally, if heavy clotting is an issue add a drop of jasmine to the mix. Because I am a cheapskate (did I mention?!) I use a jasmine maceration as the base oil instead. (Search "Jasmine Hair Oil")

2 tsp rosehip oil

Rose x 1

Clary Sage x 2

Lavender x 1

(I also like to make a little muslin bag of rose petals and ladies mantle leaves and hang it over the tap when I am running the bath!)

New Mum Bath Salts

A beautiful luxurious blend for a new mum; what shall we have? Some bath salts for those important first few baths.

We'll use rose for the feminine dimension, and to help her wound to contract. Let's add carrier and geranium to help her milk to flow nicely and reduce the milk-swelling pain in her boobs! A tiny drop of lavender for her stitches.

100g Sea Salt

Rose x 1

Geranium x 2

Carrot x 3

Lavender x 1

Wrap your jar prettily with a ribbon for a really thoughtful gift!

Post Natal Body Oil

This oil is the epitome of luxury, stuffed full of our most precious perfumery plants. A new mum can't help but feel fantastic with the oils but she will also enjoy the enhanced benefits of the bonding better with her new child.

On a more physical level, whilst we all want our figures back after that nine gruelling months of growing, growing, growing but actually it isn't that much fun when it starts to contract. For some women it can be almost as painful as giving birth was. Breast feeding will help, and so will these oils. Just be aware that some babies really don't like the "bitter taste of myrrh" when it hits the milk, so if baby starts being fussy about feeding the essential oils should be the first thing to go.

Splosh it on all over! Really hydrate the body after such an ordeal! Bliss!

100mls of rosehip oil

Rose x 1

Jasmine x 1

Celery seed x 1

Myrrh x 1

Incidentally...Don't forget there is a labour blend in my free book *The Complete Guide to Clinical Aromatherapy and the Essential Oils of the Physical Body* that was designed by Susan Mousley a former chairman of the International Federation of Aromatherapists and a midwife to boot. The blend is used on an NHS maternity ward in the East Midlands.

Breast Balm

We all need a little feminine plumping from time to time, and this is gorgeous for that, but it also specifically for breast cancer treatment patients who have suffered radiation burns from their treatments

100ml (4oz) blank moisturiser

1 tbs calendula carrier oil (or maceration, if you have them growing in the garden)

Calendula essential oil x 1

Rose x 1

Camomile matricaria x 1

Cooling Spritz

I used this in labour as well as on every hot day last summer!

Rosewater...

End of recipe!

Evaporator Oils

This is something I have become very interested in lately, mainly because I know that I am not the only therapist who is becoming increasingly distressed being asked about cures for cancer. I'll reiterate again, as yet we do not have any, but research shows that mood has a massive bearing on how well the body will heal. Not only that, but just I am a big believer in the natural order of things, is that people sadly do die. So, to me the greatest gift we can give is to help someone to have a good death. One where they feel they have answered all the questions they were here to ask and that everything they want to say can be freely told.

Emotional Holiday from Cancer

Help your loved one to switch off from fear, if only for a few moments. This is a peaceful and sensual blend, originally designed with breast cancer patients to connect better with their femininity at this time.

Use this blend in an evaporator or diffuser to soften the mood of the room.

Lemon x 3

Rose x 1

Sandalwood x 2

Bergamot x 1

Tonka bean x 1

Domestic Abuse

It is estimated that one in three women and one in six men will experience some kind of domestic abuse in their lifetime. Speaking as a survivor I know firsthand of the devastation that level of fear can leave behind.

Now we understand just how much damage that level of stress can do not only to our emotional body, but our physical body too, it is so important to find a way to lift that plaster and see what is left behind. Of course there are the *physical* scars but self esteem vanishes, lack of trust and if you are anything like I was full of self hatred. My husband gets first dibs on the excellent repair job that has done on me (and 13 years later, I'm still not really there) but rose certainly comes a close second. I have to give a hearty thanks to Marge Clarke of Nature's Gift for the idea for this blend as she was generous enough to educate me that cistus helps to remove trauma.

Rose x 1

Holy Basil x 1

Cistus x 1

Partner has left

Or actually rejection in general because I feel that is a very damaging thing to happen to someone. It is not only the primary emotion here, but the secondary ones of betrayal, anger, hatred, jealousy that begins to poison the organs.

Rose x1

Labdanum x1

Tangerine x1

Anxiety and Depression

These don't really have to have come from any particular event, I don't think. Last Thursday I woke up with a sensation of sheer dread. I had to deliberately recall each event of the previous day to try to ascertain what horror had befallen me that I should be so worried about *something*...but there was nothing. Simply chemistry that had gone a tad awry. The problems start, of course, when the chemistry becomes more permanent and this strange fearful state emerges.

A standard blend for **anxiety** might be

Rose x 1

Neroli x 1

Camomile Roman x 1

Sense of Purpose Evaporator Mix

Rose x1

Lemon x2

Bay x 1

Instil patience to wait for things to unfold

Rose x 1

Thyme x2

Benzoin x2

(I use this evaporator oil a lot when I am working on the beginning of a book and I don't know where the research will lead me)

Prayer of Gratitude

Dear God, Goddess, Divine Spirit of all there is,
Thank you for the opportunity
to gather together in one another's company.

We thank you for the light
you bring to this family gathering.

Please grant us the vision to see the highest in one another,
and grant us the opportunity to continue to be there for each other
In good times, as well as not-so-great-times.

Give us strength and fortitude to ride the tides of change,
and empower us always to be nurturing and loving with one another.

Open our spiritual eyes that we may see one another for who we truly are...
and love one other in the same spirit.

May sadness, disappointment and anger be minimal.

May happiness, positive thoughts
and good experiences together be bountiful.
May we always cope, and hope, with each other... with grace. Amen.

from A *Goddess Is A Girl's Best Friend: A Divine Guide to Finding Love,*

Success and Happiness,
By Rev Laurie Sue Brockway, Perigee Books

Conclusion

One interesting piece of information that came up during mine and Sandy's discussions about this book was that she told me that rose oil was still used today to anoint kings and queens. She described how the anointing was used to open the third eye as a mechanism to help the monarch in his wisdom for making decisions. For many days I searched and searched to try to find evidence to back this up, in fact I even drafted a letter to Prince Charles! Eventually I was able to decipher the oil she described was called Chrysm, which for the most part, is made up of myrrh. In Greek Orthodox churches, however, she is correct, the blend comprises of rose.

In my many attempts to find definitive evidence I contacted a church minister I know. He replied very quickly that he knew of an oil described in the Bible called Nard and since, in his words "Oil is just oil at the end of the day" he surmised that probably it was that that was used. (The Nard that Mary of Bethany used to anoint the Christ's feet is not rose, or chrism, it is generally accepted to be spikenard.)

Oil is just oil.... (It does make me wonder what he thinks I find to do all day)

I'm not very comfortable disagreeing with a man of the cloth, but on this point I think we have to differ!

These past three months have been extraordinary. To uncover such vast quantities of data, reiterated over and over throughout five thousand years feels like inordinate privilege. The men's sexuality research feels particularly important, not only for the wonderful medicine this can help us to give people, but also for the *scientific proof* that the physical body can be affected by the emotional aspects of our medicine too.

Because of rose, little babies have the hope of enjoying a happier first few years of life as their mommies are emotionally better equipped to take on their new role.

Mourners continue to gain blessèd relief from their grief as they absorb the tearful medicine of the hundreds of Cherokee women weeping for their loss.

Addicts will have an easier transition from dependence to sobriety, thanks to the magic of a plant. (There's a certain ironic equality that for the most part it was cannabis, poppies and hops that started their problems in the first place. Even in plant medicine we see Newton's Third Law of Motion...for every action there is an equal and opposite reaction...you just need to discover where the right plant is growing). We are only just discovering this and yet as the researchers in Greece have just uncovered... Nicolas Myrepsos knew it 800 years ago and carefully documented it in About Antidotes.

Because of rose, life lessons will be better assimilated and trauma released.

Anxiety is lifted and happiness restored.

And as for the old adage of "How many premenstrual women does it take to change a light bulb?" men may ....

No....Don't tell them! The florists need the business and I like the flowers!

So what is the roses' magic then I wonder? Is it just a sweet smelling token of love? And was my minister friend right, is oil just oil at the end of the day?

Or could it be that the feminine divine is once again exerting her might? Is she rising up and once again harnessing the energy of her sacred plant to wield her immeasurable power? Could it be that a plant will be the catalyst to release the compassionate medicine that leads us out of the Piscean age into the new enlightened and independent Age of Aquarius?

Mr Bookmaker...I'll have a fiver on rose medicine, if you please!

You may have noticed this rose book is dedicated to Suzanne, because I wanted to continue my tradition of recognising all the fans who help my cause. Su is a soap maker who uses essential oils in her darling products. You can see her clever work in the resources page. You will also find her if you visit the US reviews page where her "most helpful" review comes out on top. Very bravely she laid bare how she suspected plant medicine had helped her to overcome cancer, and the first time I read it, it made me cry.

I cried even more during writing this book, to receive a message from her to say she had a blood clot in her lungs. Regular readers of my work know I have been there, done that and wouldn't wish wearing the T-shirt on anyone. The universe seemed to be entirely against her but she has fought on, collating lists of blood thinning oils and she has made herself better! I am very proud to call her my friend. This book is to say thank you to her for her support and for her unending faith in me as a healer. Su...I am so grateful that the universe sought to finally give you a break and I fervently hope this is onwards and upwards for you.

I would also like to extend my grateful thanks to several people for their beautiful contributions to the artwork of the illustrated version of this book. Kathy Smiley of Wise Woman's Herbal (see resources) for her beautiful picture of her own rosa damascena bush from which she distils her own rose water and her enigmatic painting of the woman and her rose. To Kaja Malouf, another soap maker (again see resources) for her photos, especially my favourite one of the bees! To Robert Elsmore for his painting, but also for his unending patience with me every time he designs another one of my book covers! I am proud to extend gratitude to Neil and Pat Fletcher, my “in-laws” for the beautiful pictures of roses taken in their garden in France. A massive thank you to Sandy Humby whose rose wisdom and that of female emancipation literally leaves me gobsmacked. If you have loved the pictures she has added to the illustrated book, why not treat yourself to a pack of her enchanting golden cards to enjoy a different dimension of rose healing? (There isa lonk to her website for non-illustrated version readers to enjoy her work too)

And finally, to Lynda Jaffray, thanks for always speaking up on facebook and what turned out to be a game changing pointer of your suggestion to speak to Sandy! My next book on basil...is dedicated to you x

As ever, I feel like the book is not finished. Given the massive rose exploration in the labs, I’ll give it 12 months until it is out of date. For that reason I have pencilled in to revisit the research next year and add in further research. Ensure you are subscribed on my email list to get notification of later editions of this book and the days that you can download them for free.

You might also like to read the article that I eventually wrote for Aromatika.hu. There is nothing in it that you haven't read in this book but it is arranged in a rather amusing fashion discussing how Cleopatra used rose to get her man. I really had some fun writing it and I think reading it will probably give you a buzz.

I hope that you have enjoyed the journey as much as I have. Please do say if you like / don't like the new format with links to the trials rather than the print screens when you write your reviews. Yet again, I want to say thank you to those that have reviewed my books and have been sharing and commenting on social networks...all of those things really help me so much and I can't tell you how grateful I am.

Lastly, if you are a newcomer to my work, please also download your free copy of *The Complete Guide to Clinical Aromatherapy and The Essential Oils of the Physical Body*. It will really help you to better understand aromatherapy as an art and enable you to treat your own family simply, but more importantly safely.

So...I'm off back to the shed to write a little more about Basil (since this rose book derailed that first attempt), to enjoy the roses just starting to bloom in my own garden and also on my inevitable pilgrimage to the place I view as heaven on earth - David Austin Roses. Meanwhile, know that I am only a facebook message away. Send questions comments and, if you really must, insults to facebook.com/TheSecretHealerWrites and we'll have a good giggle together.

But for now people, to quote as the rabbit with the carrot

That's all folks!
Review and buy! Bye xxx

Resources

This book is dedicated to the lovely Suzzannemarie Bushaw, who has no idea how much she has taught me over the last few months. UK people moan continually about the state of our NHS, and none of us really has a perception of just how lucky we are to have it. Watching Su struggling with the same condition I was given free treatment for six years ago has been heart breaking for me, and I am so pleased to say she is now well.

Suzanne lives in Colorado and I absolutely love her site. I love the messages she sends me and frankly I adore *her*. Most of all though....I love her bees!

Check out her site at: http://www.beenaturalsoaps.com/

Also pop over and say hi on her two face book pages:

https://www.facebook.com/beenaturalhawaii

https://www.facebook.com/wildsoapnherbcompany

Sandy Humby

I am sure you are all aching to find more out about Sandy's beautiful meditation cards. You can find out more about both those and her extraordinary healing business at

http://www.rosealchemy.com

Kathy Smiley

What would I do without this lady? Each day she sends me lovely little stories about what is happening in her small holding. I have been thrilled to be part of her journey this year watching as she distilled rose hydrosols and made calendula macerations.

If you fancy getting something just a little bit special instead of "just rose "... if there ever could be such a thing...then pop over and see Kathy, she has magical things for sale. After a lifetime of working in herbal medicine, Kathy is about to embark into a new journey of selling in the internet.

Find her brand new website at **http://www.WildWomanHerbal.com**

Keep in touch with musings and announcements at http://www.**facebook.com/wildwomanherbal** which is one of my favourite places to hang out.

Follow her new blog at

http://www.**SmileyHolisticMedicine.com**

Kaja Malouf

Now Kaja seemed to come out of nowhere when I asked for contributors of art for the illustrated version of this book. We had never spoken before and yet she was entirely clued up on what my books were trying to do! She had been very quietly plotting, I think in the background!!!

Her pictures blew me away and her soap is utterly divine. It is lovely to be able to represent an Aussie aromatherapist here today. Here's what Kaja has to say:

I have a background in Biology with an emphasis on Anatomy and Physiology. I suffer with psoriasis and found it hard to find commercial products that didn't cause my condition to flair up. I started researching and experimenting with different oils and exfoliants. I was searching for the perfect ingredients to make my soap hydrating, good for my skin and skin condition, and of course to be simply Luscious. After testing on myself and my family I now have a goal to share my soaping experience with all. Soap making for me fulfils a life long love of Chemistry. And that's why I became a Soap maker.

We are a small scale home based company producing small batches to be able to put upmost care for every product. I prefer to sell products that are safe and mild for all skin types, sourcing local ingredients when possible, and even using organic plants we grow on our property. Kajamm products are always Palm Oil Free, often Fragrance Free (no petroleum based fragrance oils only essential oils are used), always Detergent free, and use only Natural Botanicals and Clay instead of using Synthetic Colorants. It's always been important to me to make a green product that is safe for the Environment, understanding the concept of "grey water safe".

Sustainability after all involves making choices and taking action that are in the interests of protecting the natural world so I use biodegradable packing and am always looking for better ways.

We are all responsible for the Future.

Kaja lives with her Husband and 5 Jack Russell Terriers (all rescue dogs) in a Rain Forest on the South East Coast of Australia, when she's not making soap she takes photos, plays piano, and dances with her dogs.
Kaja's beautiful website is: http://kajamm.com/pure/

She has very generously given Secret Healer readers a coupon code for 10% off all products .
Cite: **roses101**

Why not pop over and give some her artisanal products a try.

Last but certainly not least, I want to introduce you to my mom!

Jill Bruce

The Apothecary

Her knowledge of aromatherapy completely leaves mine standing. Having trained at the London School of

Aromatherapy under Patricia Davis, over 30 years ago she went on to run a very successful aromatherapy school affiliated to both the International Federation of Aromatherapy and the then International Society of Professional Aromatherapists (which is now known as IFPA.)

I trained under her and was lucky enough to serve my apprenticeship working on her travelling aromatherapy stand that visited many craft and agricultural shows each year. She is a founder member of The International Federation of Aromatherapists and you can find her shop at: https://www.etsy.com/shop/TheApothecary2

Her books **The Aura, The Garden of Eden, Out of The Labyrinth and Wicca Initiation** are available in paperback on Etsy and ebooks and paperbacks can be found on Amazon too.

Here are the rose products that *I* use (very useful to have a mum who makes rose products I can tell you!!!)

Rose and Ylang Ylang Moisturiser

Rose Gel (Which is a masque which is blissful to use and makes your skin look extraordinary!)

Rose Damask Perfume

Attar of Roses Perfume

Rose and Camellia Body Butter

And my husband swears by the **Rose Cuticle Cream** for after he has been working in the garden.

You will never find anything else to touch them, I absolutely promise.

Cover illustration and picture book layout

Robert Elsmore Images

http://robertelsmoreimages.blogspot.co.uk/

About the Author

Elizabeth Ashley qualified as an aromatherapist in 1993, and then passed her Advanced Aromatherapy Diploma in 1994. She has been practicing aromatherapy for almost 21 years.

In 1999, she fell into a whole new career in the aggressive commercial sector of recruitment consultancy. There she discovered her father's second hand car salesman genes had passed along and found she had quite a gift of the gab! More than that, she discovered she could sell…and then some.

In 2008, Elizabeth fell ill during pregnancy with a blood clot in her lungs. The pulmonary embolism prevented her from working and she started to write. Very quickly she gained her first contract as a ghost writer…a recipe book for cheese cakes!

In 2010 she was published professionally for her work on Galbanum oil in the Aromatherapy Thymes, journal of the International Federation of Aromatherapists, and on Tuberose oil by the New Zealand Register of Holistic Therapist.

In 2011 she was seconded on a consultative basis to Walsall Independent Treatment Centre, designed to be a rainbow bridge between traditional and complementary medicines. There she became aware of the rumblings of change in healthcare. Her book *Sales Strategies for Gentle Souls* explains the connotations of this.

Many of her books are aimed at helping qualified aromatherapists to expand their healing repertoire and build their businesses. She also writes for people who have an interest in essential oils and want to learn how to heal. Her in depth essential oil profiles chart the healing properties of plants from the most arcane depths of historic folklore up to the scientific lab trials of today.

In 2014 she ranks in the top 50 contract writers on the freelancer marketplace Elance.com. She is the ghost writer of seven number one Amazon best sellers in the natural healing category. She lives in Shropshire with her husband and youngest son, kept company by their cat, the budgie and many shoals of tropical fish! Her elder son and daughter attend University and make her prouder than anything ever could.

Elizabeth Ashley is possibly one of the most published aromatherapy writers you have never heard of! By 2015, all of that will have changed. Elizabeth Ashley is *The Secret Healer.*

www.thesecrethealer.co.uk

Other books in The Secret Healer Series

The Essential Oils Profiles

Monarda - A Native American Medicine

Vetiver - An Ayurvedic Medicine

Holy Basil - An Ayurvedic Medicine

The Healing Manuals

The Complete Guide to Clinical Aromatherapy & Essential Oils for the Physical Body FREE EBOOK

Book 2 Essential Oils for Mind Body Spirit

Book 3 The Essential Oil Liver Cleanse

Book 4 The Professional Stress Solution

Book 5 The Aromatherapy Eczema Treatment

Book 6 The Aromatherapy Bronchitis Treatment

Business Training for Aromatherapists

Sales Strategies for Gentle Souls

Works Cited

About Vibrational Healing. (2015). Retrieved 25 24, 2015, from Rose of Raphael.com: http://www.roseofraphael.com.au/pages/vibrational-healing

Acupuncture Today . (2015). *Rose (mei gui hua).* Retrieved 05 24, 2015, from Acupuncture Today: http://www.acupuncturetoday.com/herbcentral/rose.php

Amjad Ali, A. I. (Unlisted). *Rogane Gul - Rose Oil -A Multi potent Uniani Preparation.* Retrieved 25 24, 2015, from STM Journals : http://stmjournals.com/med/index.php?journal=AYUSH&page=article&op=view&path%5B%5D=176

Arab News. com. (2010, 12 08). *Oman's rose water: A history of tradition.* Retrieved 05 24, 2015, from Arab News.com: http://www.arabnews.com/node/362465

Bach Centre. (2009). *Wild Rose .* Retrieved 05 24, 2015, from Bach Centre.com: http://www.bachcentre.com/centre/38/wildrose.htm

Bradley BF1, S. N. (2007, 12 02). *The effects of prolonged rose odor inhalation in two animal models of anxiety.* Retrieved 05 24, 2015, from Pub med: http://www.ncbi.nlm.nih.gov/pubmed/17689573

Bruce, J. (1994). *The Garden of Eden .* Magdelena Press.

Cherokee Rose (Rosa Laevigata, Jin Ying Zi). (2012). Retrieved 05 24, 2015, from http://www.chineseherbshealing.com/cherokee-rose/: http://www.chineseherbshealing.com/cherokee-rose/

Culpepper. (n.d.). *Damask Rose .* Retrieved 05 24, 2015, from Culpeppers Complete Herbal : http://www.complete-herbal.com/culpepper/damaskrose.htm

Davis, P. (1988). *Aromatherapy and A-Z.* Saffron Waldon: C. W. Daniel Company Ltd.

de Almeida RN1, M. S. (2004, 02). *Anxiolytic-like effects of rose oil inhalation on the elevated plus-maze test in rats.* Retrieved 05 24, 2015, from Pubmed: http://www.ncbi.nlm.nih.gov/pubmed/14751465

Desert Alchemy. com. (2015). *Cliff Rose Flower Essence.* Retrieved 05 24, 2015, from https://www.desert-alchemy.com/info/flower-essence/clro/

Down, J. L. (2008). *Loving Flowers Rose Flower Essence* . Retrieved 05 24, 2015, from The Loving Feast: http://www.thehealingfeast.com/FlowerEssence.cfm

Esoteric Oils. (Unlisted). *Rosehip Oil.* Retrieved 05 24, 2015, from Esoteric Oils: http://www.essentialoils.co.za/essential-oils/rosehip.htm

Fest Flowers.com. (2015). *Green Rose.* Retrieved 05 24, 2015, from Flower Essence Services: Bridging Body and Soul: http://www.fesflowers.com/fes-store/index.php?main_page=product_info&products_id=1715

Filiberti, D. (2005). *China.* Retrieved 05 24, 2015, from Rose Gathering: http://www.rosegathering.com/china.html

Fletcher, J. (2008). *Cleopatra The Great- The Woman Behind The Legend.* London: Hodder and Stroughton.

FlowerExperty.com . (2015, 05 24). *Georgia State Flower.* Retrieved 05 24, 2015, from Flower Expert.com: http://www.theflowerexpert.com/content/aboutflowers/stateflowers/georgia-state-flowers

Flowers of India. (Unlisted). *Damask Rose.* Retrieved 25 24, 2015, from Flowers of India: http://www.flowersofindia.net/catalog/slides/Damask%20Rose.html

Fragrantica.com. (Unlisted). *Taif Rose* . Retrieved 05 24, 2015, from Fragrantica.com: http://www.fragrantica.com/notes/Taif-Rose-115.html

Goddess Guide. (2015). *Isis The Egyptian Goddess.* Retrieved 05 24, 2015, from Goddess Guide: http://www.goddess-guide.com/isis.html

Gray Crawford. (2014, 11). *Isis - The Archetype of Love and Devotion.* Retrieved 05 24, 2015, from Gray Crawford: http://graycrawford.net/2013/04/21/isis-archetype-of-love-and-devotion/

Hayward, M. (1997). *The Roses of Taif.* Retrieved 05 24, 2015, from Aramco World: https://www.saudiaramcoworld.com/issue/199706/the.roses.of.taif.htm

Herbs 2000.com. (2015). *History of The Rose.* Retrieved 05 24, 2015, from http://www.herbs2000.com/flowers/r_history.htm

Hill, J. (2010). *Isis and Ra.* Retrieved 05 24, 2015, from Gods of Ancient Egypt: http://www.ancientegyptonline.co.uk/isisra.html

Humby, S. (2015, 05 24). *Rose Alchemy.* Retrieved 05 24, 2015, from Rose Alchemy.com: http://www.rosealchemy.com/

Iles, L. (2013). *Isis, Rose of the World.* Retrieved 05 24, 2015, from Mirror of Isis: http://mirrorofisis.freeyellow.com/id125.html

Jordon, D. (2015). *Wild Rose Flower Essence The way to heal the heart.* Retrieved 05 24, 2015, from Dr Jordon.com: http://dr-jordan.com/2013/06/09/wild-rose-flower-essence-the-way-to-heal-the-heart/

Lawless, J. (1992). *The Encyclopaedia of Essential Oils.* Dorset: Element Books .

Legend ofCherokee Rose. (1996). Retrieved 05 24, 2015, from Powersource.com: http://www.powersource.com/cherokee/rose.html

Lesser, R. E. (2013, 06 12). *Rose Queen of Flowers - Secret Healer* . Retrieved 05 24, 2015, from Ruth E Lesser: https://ruthelsesser.wordpress.com/2013/06/12/rose-queen-of-flowers-sacred-healer/

Making Rose Sugar. (2014, 04 24). Retrieved 05 24, 2015, from The Charm of Home Blogspot : http://thecharmofhome.blogspot.co.uk/2012/04/making-rose-sugar.html

Manniche, L. (1989). *An Egyptian Herbal* . London: British Museum Press.

manniche, L. (1999). *Sacred Luxuries;Fragrance, Aromatherapy and Cosmetics in Ancient Egypt.* London: Opus Publishing.

Marina. (2015). *ROSES IN GREEK HISTORY, CULTURE AND MYTHOLOGY.* Retrieved 05 24, 2015, from Yummy Cyprus:

http://www.yummycyprus.com/index.cfm/id/news/lang/english/page/2/type/121/recID/1724/Roses_in_Greek_history,_culture_and_mythology

Mojay, G. (1996). *Aromatherapy for Healing the Spirit: Restoring Emotional and Mental Balance with Essential Oils.* Tankabon.

Morrison Gardens. (2014). *The Meaning of Rose Colours.* Retrieved 05 24, 2015, from http://www.rkdn.org/roses/colors.asp

Natural Home Remedy . (2015). *Natural Home Remedy - Rose Centifolia.* Retrieved 05 25, 2015, from Natural Home Remedy : http://naturalhomeremedies.co/Rose.html

Nazıroğlu M1, K. S. (2013, 01). *Rose oil (from Rosa × damascena Mill.) vapor attenuates depression-induced oxidative toxicity in rat brain.* Retrieved 05 24, 2015, from Pubmed: http://www.ncbi.nlm.nih.gov/pubmed/22484603

nmessences.com. (2015). *Yellow Rose.* Retrieved 05 24, 2015, from http://www.nmessences.com/essences/rose_yel_trauma.html

Oman Info. (2011, 03 09). *Roses bring scent of success to highlands.* Retrieved 05 24, 2015, from Oman Info: http://www.omaninfo.com/news/roses-bring-scent-success-highlands.asp

Rich, P. (1994). *Practical Aromatherapy.* London: Paragon .

Rose . (n.d.). Retrieved 05 24, 2015, from Wikepedia: http://en.wikipedia.org/wiki/Rose

Rose and Cardomom Porrige. (Unlisted). Retrieved 05 24, 2015, from Psychologies: https://psychologies.co.uk/rose-cardamom-pistachio-porridge

Rose Cottage Flower Essences. (2015). *Rose Essences.* Retrieved 05 24, 2015, from Unfolding Enlightenment.com: http://www.unfoldingenlightenment.com/RoseCottageFlowerEssences/index.html

Rose Essence . (2015). Retrieved 05 24, 2015, from Floracopeia: http://www.floracopeia.com/Flower-Essences/Rose-Flower-Essence.html

Rose Flower Essence . (2015). Retrieved 05 24, 2015, from Still point aromatics: http://www.stillpointaromatics.com/alchemystical-apothecary-rose-flower-essence-love

Sachs, M. (1994). *Ayurvedic Beauty Care.* Twin Lakes Wisconsin: Lotus Books.

Sacred Lotus. (2015). *Chinese Herb: Mei Gui Hua (Young Flower of Chinese Rose (Bud)), Flos Rosae Rugosae.* Retrieved 05 24, 2015, from Sacred Lotus: http://www.sacredlotus.com/go/chinese-herbs/substance/mei-gui-hua-young-flower-of-chinese-rose-bud

Schmitt S, S. U. (2010). Variation of in vitro human skin permeation of rose oil between different application sites. *Komplementarmedizin* .

Schotte, N. (2015). *Flower Essences.* Retrieved 05 24, 2015, from La Vie De La Rose: https://laviedelarose.com/

Semiata-Akuaba, T. (2003). *Rose Flower Essences: loving Support Through Life's Transitions.* Retrieved 05 24, 2015, from Flower Essence Magazine.com: http://www.floweressencemagazine.com/feb03/roseessences.html

T, H. (2009). Relaxing effect of rose oil on human. *Natural Product Communications* .

The Meanings of Rose Colours. (2015). Retrieved 05 24, 2015, from Rose for Love.com: http://www.roseforlove.com/the-meanings-of-rose-colors-ezp-22

The Perfume Society . (2015). *The Romans: when fountains flowed with rosewater.* Retrieved 05 24, 2015, from The Perfume Society : http://perfumesociety.org/discover-perfume/an-introduction/history/the-romans-when-rosewater-flowed-through-fountains/

Tisserand, R. (1988). *Aromatherapy for Everyone.* London: Penguin Books.

Tisserand, R. (1977). *The Art of Aromatherapy.* Saffron Walden : The C. W Daniel Company Limited.

Trade India. (n.d.). *Rose Absolute* . Retrieved 05 24, 2015, from Trade India: http://www.tradeindia.com/fp501360/ROSE-ABSOLUTE-RUH-GULAB-.html

Tree Frog Farm. (2015). *Nootka Wild FlowerEssence* . Retrieved 05 24, 2015, from Tree Frog Farm: http://www.treefrogfarm.com/store/flower-essences-tree-essences/nootka-wild-rose-flower-essence.html

White Rose Aromatics. (2009, 09 03). *White Rose Aromatics.* Retrieved 05 24, 2015, from Ruh Gulab/Rose otto(Rosa damascena) essential oil/Himalayas, India organic: http://www.whitelotusblog.com/2009/09/ruh-gulabrose-ottorosa-damascena.html

Why the Rose Balances the Heart. (2015). Retrieved 24 05, from maharishi Ayurveda: http://www.mapi.com/ayurvedic-knowledge/personal-goals/balance-the-heart-with-roses-and-ayurveda.html

Wildwood, C. (1996). *The Encyclopoeadia of Aromatherapy.* London: BloomsburyPublishing.

Worwood, V. A. (1987). *Aromantics.* Great Britain: Bantam Books.

Yin Yan House- Theory. (2015). *Jin Ying Zi (Cherokee Rosehip) - Chinese Herbal Medicine.* Retrieved 05 24, 2015, from https://theory.yinyanghouse.com/theory/herbalmedicine/jin_ying_zi_tcm_herbal_database

Aghsane. (2013). *Rose OIl.* Retrieved 05 19, 2015, from Export Markets.com: http://aghsane_2.exportmarkets.com/product/20345/rose-oil

Case Study Summary: BULGARIAN ROSE OIL. (Unlisted). Retrieved 05 19, 2015, from Ecologic.de: http://www.ecologic.de/download/projekte/1800-1849/1802/rose_oil.pdf

Dawn. (2006, 02 06). *Essential Oil Extraction from Roses.* Retrieved 05 19, 2015, from Dawn.com: http://www.dawn.com/news/177445/essential-oil-extraction-from-roses

Eans, D. (2015). *Essential Oils of Rose - Wisdom of Arabia.* Retrieved 05 19, 2015, from Herbal Educator.com: http://herbaleducator.com/essential-oil-of-rose-wisdom-of-arabia/

Enio Bonchev. (2015). *History of Bulgarian Rose.* Retrieved 05 19, 2015, from Enio Bonchev: http://www.eniobonchev.com/en/history/

European Cities Past and Present. (2015). *Rose and Rose Production .* Retrieved 05 19, 2015, from European Cities Past And Present: https://europeancitiespastandpresent.wikispaces.com/Rose+and+rose+oil+production?responseToken=1ed0904f8c3cc0f5bb224f857ead776b

Focus Fen. (2012, 05 05). *Prof. Nedko Nedkov: About 99% of rose oil produced in Bulgaria is exported.* Retrieved 05 19, 2015, from Planet Radio: http://www.focus-fen.net/opinion/0000/00/00/2879/

Fukada M, K. E. (2011, 10 30). *Effect of "rose essential oil" inhalation on stress-induced skin-barrier disruption in rats and humans.* Retrieved 05 15, 2015, from Aromatic Science: https://www.aromaticscience.com/effect-of-rose-essential-oil-inhalation-on-stress-induced-skin-barrier-disruption-in-rats-and-humans-2/

Gholamhoseinian A1, F. H. (2009, 10 16). *Inhibitory effect of methanol extract of Rosa damascena Mill. flowers on alpha-glucosidase activity and postprandial hyperglycemia in normal and diabetic rats.* Retrieved 05 15, 2015, from Pubmed: http://www.ncbi.nlm.nih.gov/pubmed/19380218

Grieve, M. M. (2014). *Roses.* Retrieved 05 19, 2015, from Botanica.com: http://www.botanical.com/botanical/mgmh/r/roses-18.html

Han SH1, H. M. (2006, 07). *Effect of aromatherapy on symptoms of dysmenorrhea in college students: A randomized placebo-controlled clinical trial.* Retrieved 05 15, 2015, from Pubmed: http://www.ncbi.nlm.nih.gov/pubmed/16884344

Journey to the Rose Country. (2015). Retrieved 05 19, 2015, from Biolandes: http://www.biolandes.com/en-voyage-to-the-country-of-rose.php?voyage=o&lg=en

Mika Fukada1, 2. E. (2011, 10 30). *Effect of "Rose Essential Oil" Inhalation on Stress-Induced Skin-Barrier Disruption in Rats and Humans.* Retrieved 05 19, 2015, from Oxford Journals.org: http://chemse.oxfordjournals.org/content/37/4/347.long

Nazıroğlu M1, K. S. (213, 01). *Rose oil (from Rosa × damascena Mill.) vapor attenuates depression-induced oxidative toxicity in rat brain.* Retrieved 05 19, 2015, from Pubmed: http://www.ncbi.nlm.nih.gov/pubmed/22484603

P, C., & C, A. (2012, 06 12). *The effects of clinical aromatherapy for anxiety and depression in the high risk postpartum woman – A pilot study.* Retrieved 05 15,

2015, from Aromatic Science: http://www.ctcpjournal.com/article/S1744-3881(12)00040-0/abstract

Pappas, R. (2015). *Rose.* Retrieved 05 19, 2015, from Essential Oil University : http://essentialoil.university/search/index?q=rose

S. Taavoni, F. D. (2013, 04 18). *The effect of aromatherapy massage on the psychological symptoms of postmenopausal Iranian women.* Retrieved 050 15, 2015, from Complementary Therapies in medicine: http://www.complementarytherapiesinmedicine.com/article/S0965-2299(13)00062-9/abstract

Sadeghi Aval Shahr H1, S. M. (2014, 09). *The effect of self-aromatherapy massage of the abdomen on the primary dysmenorrhoea.* Retrieved 05 015, 2015, from Pubmed: http://www.ncbi.nlm.nih.gov/pubmed/25254570

The Rose of Taif. (n.d.). Retrieved 05 19, 2015, from Aramco World: https://www.saudiaramcoworld.com/issue/199706/the.roses.of.taif.htm

Turkey: Rose and Other Essential Oils. (Unlisted). Retrieved 05 15, 2015, from ITC trade Impact for Good: http://www.intracen.org/uploadedFiles/intracenorg/Content/Exporters/Market_Data_and_Information/Market_information/Market_Insider/Essential_Oils/Turkey%20and%20Rose%20Oil.pdf

Why Rose Balances The Heart. (2014). Retrieved 05 19, 2015, from Mapi.com: http://www.mapi.com/ayurvedic-knowledge/personal-goals/balance-the-heart-with-roses-and-ayurveda.html

Yu Ri Kim, 1. J.-H.-J. (2014, 11 26). *Clinical Evaluation of a New-Formula Shampoo for Scalp Seborrheic Dermatitis Containing Extract of Rosa centifolia Petals and Epigallocatechin Gallate: A Randomized, Double-Blind, Controlled Study.* Retrieved 05 15, 2015, from Pubmed: http://www.ncbi.nlm.nih.gov/pmc/articles/PMC4252671/

Disclaimer

by SEQ Legal

(1) Introduction

This disclaimer governs the use of this book. [By using this book, you accept this disclaimer in full. / We will ask you to agree to this disclaimer before you can access the book.]

(2) Credit

This disclaimer was created using an SEQ Legal template.

(3) No advice

The book contains information about aromatherapy and the use of essential oils.The information is not advice, and should not be treated as such.

[You must not rely on the information in the book as an alternative to qualified medical advice from a health professional. advice from an appropriately qualified professional. If you have any specific questions about any medical matter you should consult an appropriately qualified professional.]

[If you think you may be suffering from any medical condition you should seek immediate medical attention. You should never delay seeking medical advice, disregard medical advice, or discontinue medical treatment because of information in the book.]

(4) No representations or warranties

To the maximum extent permitted by applicable law and subject to section 6 below, we exclude all representations, warranties, undertakings and guarantees relating to the book.

Without prejudice to the generality of the foregoing paragraph, we do not represent, warrant, undertake or guarantee:

> that the information in the book is correct, accurate, complete or non-misleading;
>
> that the use of the guidance in the book will lead to any particular outcome or result; or
>
> in particular, that by using the guidance in the book you will heal disease or work in any way as a cure for illness.

(5) Limitations and exclusions of liability

The limitations and exclusions of liability set out in this section and elsewhere in this disclaimer: are subject to section 6 below; and govern all liabilities arising under the disclaimer or in relation to the book, including liabilities arising in contract, in tort (including negligence) and for breach of statutory duty.

We will not be liable to you in respect of any losses arising out of any event or events beyond our reasonable control.

We will not be liable to you in respect of any business losses, including without limitation loss of or damage to profits, income, revenue, use, production, anticipated savings, business, contracts, commercial opportunities or goodwill.

We will not be liable to you in respect of any loss or corruption of any data, database or software.

We will not be liable to you in respect of any special, indirect or consequential loss or damage.

(6) Exceptions

Nothing in this disclaimer shall: limit or exclude our liability for death or personal injury resulting from negligence; limit or exclude our liability for fraud or fraudulent misrepresentation; limit any of our liabilities in any way that is not permitted under applicable law; or exclude any of our liabilities that may not be excluded under applicable law.

(7) Severability

If a section of this disclaimer is determined by any court or other competent authority to be unlawful and/or unenforceable, the other sections of this disclaimer continue in effect.

If any unlawful and/or unenforceable section would be lawful or enforceable if part of it were deleted, that part will be deemed to be deleted, and the rest of the section will continue in effect.

(8) Law and jurisdiction

This disclaimer will be governed by and construed in accordance with English law, and any disputes relating to this disclaimer will be subject to the exclusive jurisdiction of the courts of England and Wales.

(9) Our details

In this disclaimer, "we" means (and "us" and "our" refer to) [*Build Your Own Reality)*] of [*SY8 1LQ)*].

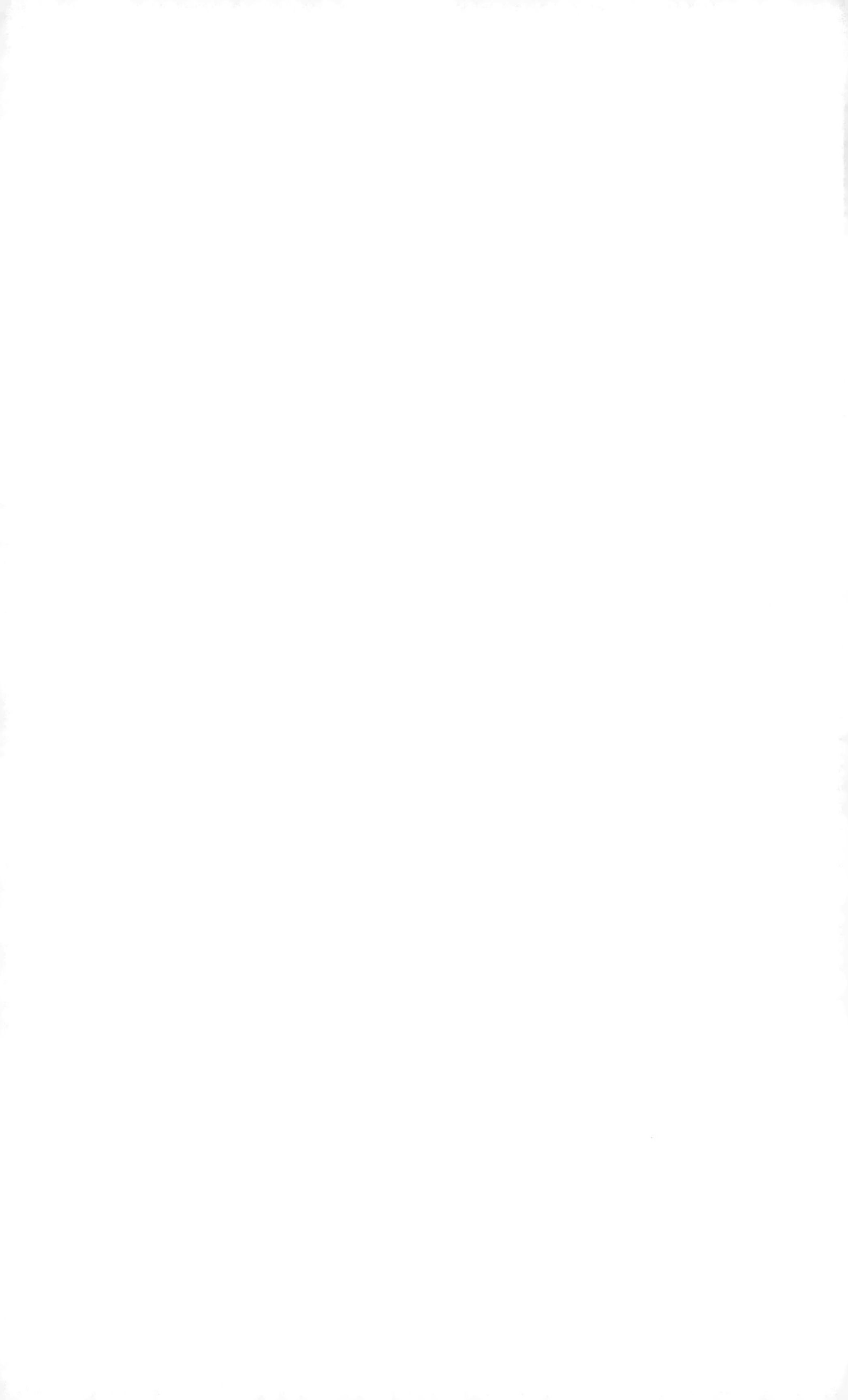

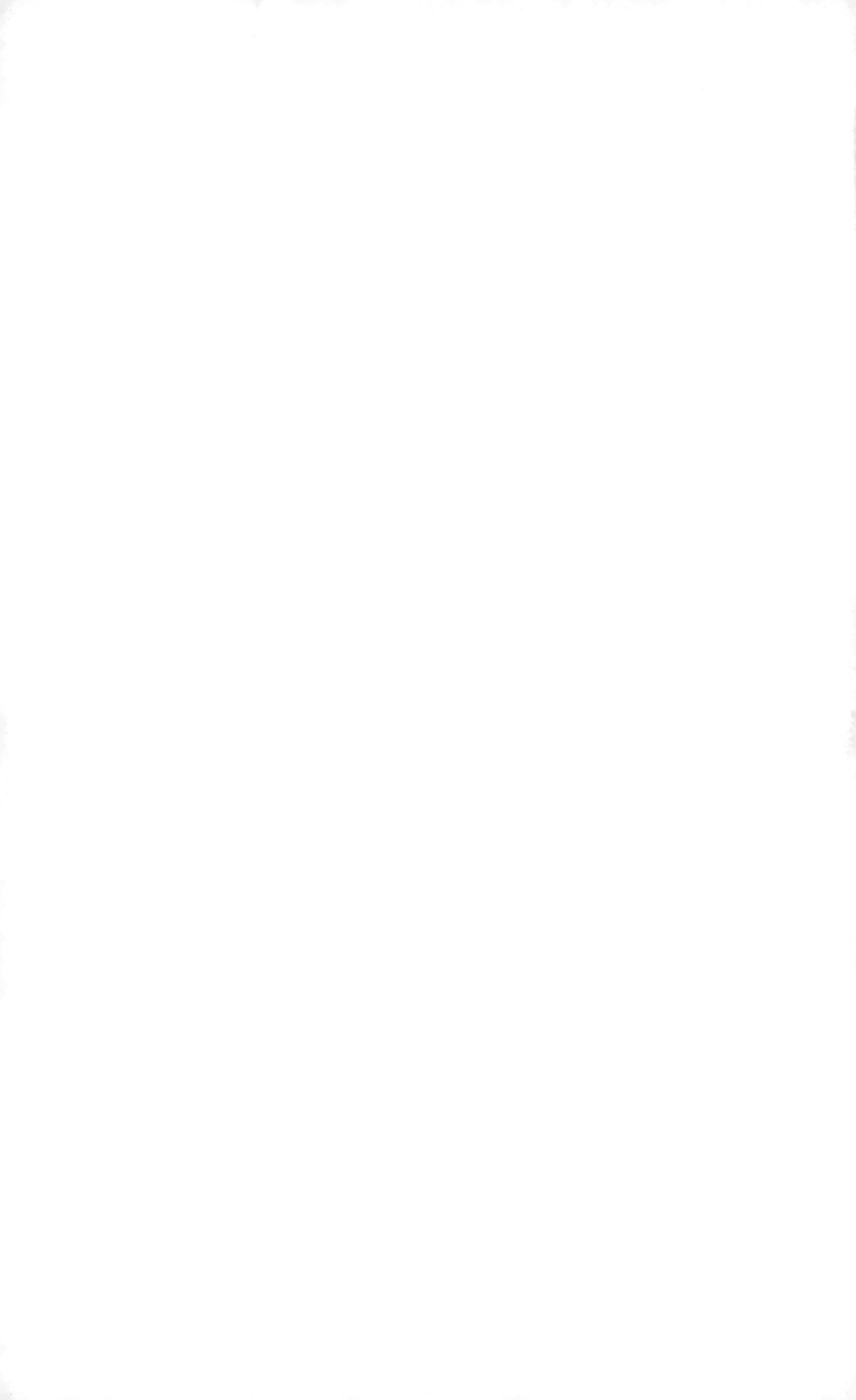

www.ingramcontent.com/pod-product-compliance
Ingram Content Group UK Ltd.
Pitfield, Milton Keynes, MK11 3LW, UK
UKHW020144250726
13967UKWH00002B/861